A LITTLE LIFE IN YOU YET

How I Beat 10 Years of Infertility for $20

HENGIST MOUNTEBANK

A LITTLE LIFE IN YOU YET
Copyright © 2019

All Rights Reserved

No part of this book may be reproduced, stored in a retrieval system, or transmitted in any form or by any means, electronic, mechanical, photocopying, recording, scanning, or otherwise, without the prior written permission of the publisher.

Contents

Introduction --- 1

Chapter 1: How I Became A Mountebank --- 11

Chapter 2: Infertility --- 33

Chapter 3: Eureka! --- 45

Chapter 4: Eureka Explained For Massive Dummies Like Me --- 47

Chapter 5: For The Truly And Hopelessly Dense --- 53

Chapter 6: Science Stuff --- 57

Chapter 7: Safety Stuff --- 67

Chapter 8: The Great Day --- 77

Chapter 9: Matilda Is Born --- 83

Chapter 10: Calamity --- 85

Chapter 11: Florentina Is Born --- 93

Chapter 12: Conclusion --- 101

Chapter 13: Your Baker's Dozen --- 105

Chapter 14: Volunteer Study --- 111

Afterword --- 116

INTRODUCTION

There are couples who can be happy and fulfilled without children, and there are couples who cannot. My wife and I could not. We wanted a child with all our hearts. We desperately needed a child. But we couldn't make one. The doctors couldn't make one from us, either, in spite of all their trying. And so my wife and I were like that lady in the Bible who "suffered many things of many physicians, and had spent all that she had, and was nothing bettered, but rather grew worse." That was us.

For ten years I prayed, and never stopped. No, that's a lie. Of course I sometimes stopped. I rage quit. But I always came back again, and got back to praying again. That is true.

Finally, it came to me. An idea. Whether it came from God directly, or whether it bubbled up out of my own brain, I don't know. I'm inclined to believe the former. And now I am going to tell you this idea. No, I'm not going to tease you and keep it for later in the book. I'm going to tell it to you right here, right now. Because if *you* are dealing with infertility, I know the value of your time.

Here was my idea.

"Saturate your testicles with dimethyl sulfoxide."

There you go. There's your price of admission, right there. And now, if *you* want to go and saturate *your* testicles with dimethyl sulfoxide - or the testicles of someone you love - you can close this book, and go do that. Bye! Good luck!

For those of you remaining - and I hope someone's still here I will tell you the whole story of how my wife and I overcame a decade of infertility to get two healthy, funny, smart, beautiful daughters.

Let me just say first, this is not advice. I'm telling you what I did, and how it worked out wonderfully and miraculously for my wife and me. You should do whatever you think is good for your family and yourself; and that's the only advice I have for you, my friend.

I call you friend because I feel like I know you. Let me see. You feel like you want to give up. You're sick of the struggle, sick of living, sick of it all. You blame yourself. You're afraid. You're lonely. You feel like a loser. Your marriage is hurting. Pregnancy/birth announcements make you sad. Or mad. You get jealous of your friends, jealous of your relatives, and you hate yourself for that. Infertility is hell.

One hard part of infertility is that nobody wants to talk about it. Everyone avoids it like something dirty on the sidewalk. Everyone feels awkward and ashamed. I did too. But now I have this hopeful story, so I'm sharing it with everyone I can.

Quick summary, just so you know what you're in for. I saturated my testicles, actually my whole dickenballs, with dimethyl sulfoxide. Almost immediately, my wife conceived our first child, a perfect baby girl. My beautiful, darling, wonderful Matilda. After ten years of nothing.

We had a postpartum complication. Because of this, and because of our ages, the doctors told us, "No more babies."

No problem there, we thought. No more babies? That's the easiest thing in the world! We were, up until now, the world champions of not making babies!

I put the dimethyl sulfoxide away, and never used it again. At least, not on the old meat and two veg. We were perfectly satisfied, anyway, with just Matilda. One child is about a million billion trillion times better than none.

Then oops, I made my wife pregnant again. Whatever miracle dimethyl sulfoxide had worked, it had apparently worked for good. Another anxious pregnancy, and another perfect, wonderful, darling baby girl: Florentina.

More warnings from our doctors. "Really, no more children!" So we're done. A happy family of four. After ten years wandering in the infertility wilderness, we've reached our Promised Land. We spent a hell of a lot of money on impotent doctors. Sometimes it felt like the ordeal of infertility might cost us our marriage, too. In the end, the solution was a $20 bottle of dimethyl sulfoxide I bought on the internet. On eBay! So that's your risk if you try to copy me, twenty dollars. Well, 20 bucks plus the cost of this book.

What about safety? That's all in Chapter Seven, but I will tell you this much now. Dimethyl sulfoxide has been well studied for over 100 years, including extensive toxicology testing on humans. In the opinion of Dr. Morton Walker, who wrote a whole book on the subject, dimethyl sulfoxide is safer than sugar. It is safer than salt. It is safer than coffee and tea.

What is my agenda? I don't sell dimethyl sulfoxide. I don't own stocks in it. I am writing and selling this book, but I could have written other books. For example, "How to Regrow a Mutilated Nose." But I'm going to give you that story too, in Chapter Thirteen, for a bonus.

My agenda does have a few items on it, however. First, I want to help other couples to find their way out of infertility. I want you to be parents. I want you to have fulfilment and joy.

Second, I want to help the babies. I want them to be born. I want them to love and be loved. I want them to be loved by you.

Third, I cannot not-write this book. If I just sat on what I know, I'd be as bad as someone sitting on a cure for cancer. In some ways, I'd be worse. Withholding a cure for cancer would deny people years of life, and years of loving relationships. Withholding *my* discovery could deny people life, period. It could deny them love, period. Relationships, period. I don't want to answer to God for that.

I am only too aware that this book may come too late for someone. First, because I did put off writing it for a few years. Partly because I wanted to be sure that our own little guinea pigs were totally healthy and normal.

They are. Both of our girls are healthy, robust, intelligent, and hilarious.

I also put off writing this because, well, I felt that someone else should have written it. Someone with initials after his name. Someone with a lab coat, and a comb-over, and file cabinets crammed with meticulous data. Someone who has done random double-blind studies, and all of that. It shouldn't be left to a no-name kook like me. I'm not a famous doctor like Dr. T.

Doctor T!

The medical profession and I don't always get along, but Dr. T. is a very special exception. He is one of the top men in his area of speciality. One of the top men in the world. This is not an exaggeration. I have seen the rankings, and he is really ranked that highly.

He is a brilliant, dedicated physician. He loves his patients. He tells me when he loses one, and sometimes he cries. Every doctor cannot be the top man in his field, but in a perfect world every doctor would have the devotion and compassion of Dr. T.

Additionally, Dr. T. is good talker, a bon vivant, and - one of my best friends. Next week he is coming over for a barbecue. We're doing beef cheeks braised in red wine. While that's cooking, (about 4 hours) Dr. T. and I will be having some beers, and shooting the breeze, and playing with my daughters. Other children from the neighbourhood will pop by, and we will feed them hot dogs.

Frankly, I envy Dr. T. because he is rich and famous and professionally accomplished. But Dr. T. frankly envies *me* because I have a loving family in a happy home. Dr. T. wanted a family of his own, but he always prioritized his research and his patients. So he likes to hang out with us, and we love to have him.

Well, I called up Dr. T. and asked him to come to my office, and not bring his car. After he arrived I opened a nice Scotch whisky I'd been saving, and sat down with Dr. T., and told him my story. *This* story. How I got Matilda and Florentina, with the help of dimethyl sulfoxide.

Dr. T. listened carefully. He questioned me, and I also questioned him. We talked for about two hours. In the end I asked him. Was it at least possible that it was the dimethyl sulfoxide that fixed our infertility? Or was I crazy?

Dr. T. said, "No, Hengist, you are not crazy. Your theory is excellent. (Ingenious, amazing, and a miracle are other words he used.) And it worked. It seems clear to me that you are right."

I asked him if it would be irresponsible of me, or unethical, or illegal, or bad, to tell infertile people what I did.

Dr. T. said, "No. That would not be a bad thing. It would be a good thing. You might help a lot of people. You should do it!"

We talked about safety. Dr. T. reassured me that using dimethyl sulfoxide, in the way that I did, is perfectly safe.

"You think I should write this book?"

"Yes."

It is therefore with my friend's blessing that I present this little book. Any mistakes are mine alone, and I'm sorry. I'm just a layman and a dummy and a mountebank. You and I both could wish that this book had been written for us by a qualified medical professional. As Dr. T points out, however, a qualified medical professional would be very unlikely to write it. They don't like being laughed at.

And so, great burdens fall sometimes on fat little hobbits like me. If anyone else has made this same discovery independently, get in touch with me. We'll name the technique after *you*, and we'll nominate *you* for the Nobel Prize, and we'll split the cash. I am not out to steal anyone's thunder or glory. But a*s far as Dr. T. and I know*, I am the first person, and still the only person, to come up with this cheap, safe, and (in my case) effective fix to infertility.

Besides not being a scientist or physician, I am also not a professional writer. And I'm not very professional in general. Please bear with me. Especially when we come to my silly little farce about Chad. But anyway, I wrote the damn book. It took me a couple of drafts, but here it is.

More time was lost offering it to publishers. No one wanted to touch it. Well, I can't blame them. If I were a respectable publisher, I wouldn't touch this book with a ten-foot barge pole. A compilation of anecdotes by some obscure crank? Talking about dunking your nuts in an industrial solvent? So I decided to publish it by myself.

More time got lost communicating with YouTube celebrities. "What good will it do to self-publish my book," I thought, when no one knows or cares who I am? Before self-publishing, it would be a good idea to generate some sort of demand.

I typed "infertility" into YouTube, and sent emails to all of the channels that have addressed the topic. Not all, but as many as had a substantial audience, which I considered to be in the high hundreds.

I never got any replies.

Not one channel wrote back a single rejection.

"Well, Hengist Mountebank," I said to myself. "Like the Little Red Hen, you are going to have to do this ALL BY YOURSELF."

So I made a YouTube channel, and called it, "Hengist Mountebank Presents." In two months the audience grew to 20,000 subscribers, and I was making money. As much as two hundred dollars a day! In three months, YouTube demonetized me. That's okay, YouTube. You can demonetize me, but you cannot demoralize me. My videos were always, from the beginning, to find an audience for this book. Babies will be born, parents will be made, marriages will be saved because of it. That is a million billion trillion times more valuable than your advertising revenue.

So here we are, after many bumps and potholes and deadend alleyways and flat tires.

One more time, this book is not advice. It makes no claims or guarantees. If I *do* get too excited, and if I *do* give you advice, or claims, or guarantees, please disregard them. I accept no liability or complaints or bad attention of any kind.

On the other hand, if you want to contact me with questions, comments, criticisms, or what-have-you, please do! You can find my email address at the end of the book.

If you decide, by and for yourself, to emulate my technique, then I strongly urge you to contact me and join my open study. That is described in Chapter Fourteen.

And if you would like to shoot me a tip, you can also find my donation links there. Hey, I'm not ashamed to suggest it. Maybe this information saves you a lot of doctor bills, and maybe you'd like to toss me a small part of the money I've helped you to save! Self-published cranks like me get no publisher's advance, remember. This book has been 100% funded by me, in time diverted from my own business. And by my family, in time diverted from them. Okay, that's enough of that. Please donate or not, as you feel guided.

My title is from the song *This Woman's Work*, by the great Kate Bush. The full line is, "I know you've got a little life in you yet." I believe this for you, Reader. I would never raise your hopes unless I believed it with all my heart. And this is what makes me so confident: I have the best evidence.

My evidence is upstairs, sleeping peacefully in their little beds.

1
HOW I BECAME A MOUNTEBANK

I will tell you how I became a mountebank, but first I must tell you what a mountebank is, and why I chose the name. From the Oxford Dictionary:

Mountebank: An itinerant quack who from an elevated platform appealed to his audience by means of stories, tricks, juggling, and the like, in which he was often assisted by a professional clown or fool.

And:

Quack: An ignorant pretender to medical or surgical skill; one who boasts to have a knowledge of wonderful remedies; an empiric or imposter in medicine.

Some people mistakenly think that the words mountebank, and quack, are synonymous with charlatan, fraudster, hoaxter, trickster, swindler, cheater, hoodwinker, confidence man. This is false. As we can see from these dictionary definitions, a mountebank, or a quack, may be perfectly honest and well-intentioned. As, I assure you, I am.

Furthermore, I am honestly ignorant of medicine. I am a medical ignoramus. But an ignoramus is not always wrong. An ignoramus can be right. I think I'm right, and my wife thinks I'm right, and my children think I'm right, and their grateful grandparents think I'm right. And my friend, Dr. T., thinks I'm right.

Also, I knew that people were going to call me a mountebank anyway, along with a quack, and a kook, and everything else. So why not own it? I feel like a mountebank when I say to another man (or woman), "Here's my miracle cure. Now what you do is, you rub this stuff all over your balls and ovaries!" I do have some self-awareness, you know. Does that message sound preposterous to you? Then imagine how much it feels preposterous to me. But what else can I do? This is the only cure for infertility that I have, and I can't stay silent about it forever.

Also, I am Canadian, and if there is one thing Canadians know how to do, it is to deprecate themselves. Oh sorry, two things. Canadians know two things. Self-deprecation and apologies.

Also, I think it just sounds funny and nice in itself: Hengist Mountebank. It is romantic and dashing.

Also, YouTube is our modern-day equivalent of the raised platform. I try to fill my channel with badly-drawn cartoons in an attempt to gain an audience. As many as possible. Because according to Wikipedia, twenty percent of them are going to be infertile. So I am very much acting the part of a mountebank. But I have no assistants. I have to be mountebank, clown, and fool, all in one.

I don't mind playing the fool, just as Saint Paul wasn't ashamed to be a fool for the sake of the Gospel. Not to compare myself too directly with Saint Paul, you know, despite the obvious parallels. He didn't plan on becoming an apostle of the gospel; I didn't plan on becoming the apostle of rubbing dimethyl sulfoxide on your balls. He endured ridicule and stonings, and eventually beheading; I endure ridicule and down thumbs and channel demonetization. That's all I'm saying.

Hey, I wish a better, easier, more comfortable and respectable route were available. It would be great if I could just go to a medical conference, stand at a podium, and deliver my hypothesis, and my testing, and my results. If they ever invite me, sure, I'll go. I'll go anywhere in the world! In the meantime, making humorous videos on YouTube is the best way I could think of to gather a crowd.

Finally, I didn't use my real-life name because the information in here is so personal. This is my health and reproductive history. And not only mine. It's my wife's health and reproductive history. And it's my children's history, too. It's private stuff - that I have to make as public as possible.

I don't know my OpSec from my elbow. I'm probably easy to dox. To anyone thinking about doing that, I'm asking you nicely. Please don't. It wouldn't even hurt me so much, but it would hurt my wife. And that would hurt me. I'm sticking my neck out here, and trusting in human kindness. Please don't step on my neck.

All right, that explains what a mountebank is, and why I wear the name. Now for how I actually became one.

Circumstances made me a mountebank. I had been married about a year when I came home one night and found my wife in tears.

"My dad has cancer."

It was lung cancer, and one of the nastier kinds. The 5-year survival rate for my father-in-law was about 7 percent.

They took out one of his lungs, and half of the other. If you do the math, that left the poor man with only a quarter of his original lung capacity. But it was enough. As soon as he recovered, he went right back to farming. He farmed as hard as ever. "All's well that ends well," we thought. Then my wife mentioned something the doctor had said. Something that made me furious and drove me on my one-way trip down Mountebank Lane. What did the doctor say?

He said: "You'd better not get lung cancer again, or there's nothing I can do for you."

Imagine that. You are a highly paid, highly privileged medical man. The world's knowledge is at your fingertips. You have libraries and archives of resources not available to the common man. You have colleagues to consult. You could write to the finest specialists in the world. You have, presumably, taken some sort of oath to your patients. But there's nothing you can do. Oh, really. You cannot help. You cannot try. The real truth is, we both know, you cannot be bothered.

I have a love-hate relationship with the medical profession. Dr. T. represents the love side, and this lazy, heartless man represents the hate side. Someone with duty, credentials, training, vows, the public trust, public investment, everything, says, "Nothing I can do."

Fine, is my answer to people like him. Thanks, at least, for letting us know we can't rely on you.

"If this man doesn't want to do his job," I told my wife. "If he won't do his job, I should say, then I'll do it for him."

"What do you mean?"

"There must be some therapies or something. Home remedies. We'll find them. I'll find them."

"But how will you…"

"The internet!"

So I became an internet health kook, the kind who pesters you on all your social media. I read everything I could about diets, supplements, treatments. Every week new books, gadgets, bottles of pills, and bags of herbs arrived at our house. I was spending all of our money. I also sought out local plants and made my own concoctions and decoctions.

Father-in-law received some things kindly. Others he kindly refused. That was his business, and I tried never to push anything too hard. It was my job to learn, and to be lab rat #1, and offer ideas. Never to push.

In recent years I have learned that I am a direct descendant of the great French pioneer to New France, and comrade of Samuel Champlain - the apothecary, Louis Hébert. But I did not know this at the time. At the time, I drew inspiration was my mother. To be specific, I was inspired by the time that she healed me, once, of what I took to be a deadly case of knee cancer.

I have always been a raging hypochondriac. Combine this with a morbid fascination for the Reader's Digest's Drama in Real Life features. Remember those? Little girl develops a pimple. Pimple grows. Turns out it's flesh-eating disease, and the girl loses her limbs. Horrible stories like that. And then, of course, to a kid like me, every pimple is probably going to turn into flesh-eating disease. I must have read one of those stories about breast cancer. And the breast cancer must have started out as a lump. Because when I was was seven when I got a lump on my knee, and I knew that it had to be knee cancer.

That was too scary to deal with, so I wore long pants and tried to ignore it. The cancer grew. I could hardly put my pants on anymore. At last, one night it was too big and painful to ignore any longer. I brought it to my mother.

"It's probably not knee cancer, Hengist," she said.

"I beg to disagree, Mother," I said.

"Let's get Mrs. Simpson's opinion."

Mrs. Simpson was a nurse. She lived next door.

"Oh, that's just a boil. Looks pretty painful, right? It's got to be lanced. Bring him to the clinic in the morning."

So my mom was right. It wasn't knee cancer after all. Phew. But my relief was short-lived. When Mrs. Simpson had gone, I asked my mom what lancing was. She told me, and I almost passed out.

"Well, if you don't want to lance it, I suppose we could try plantain."

"What's that? Does it hurt?"

Plantain is a plant, my mother explained. A common weed. If we could find some plantain and mash it up, my mom would put the mash on my knee, and wrap it up with a bandage, and put me to bed. In the morning, my boil might be gone. But if it was still there, we would get it lanced.

My dad went out with a flashlight to look for plantain in our yard. He found some. My mom mashed it up and put it on my knee. I went to bed. In the morning, we unwrapped it.

The boil was completely gone.

"Look here," said my mom, showing me inside the bandage. The dark green mash was covered with yellowish ooze. The plantain had sucked out all the pus.

That experience taught me that you don't always have to listen to your good-for-nothing doctor when he tells you that there's "nothing he can do." You don't always just have to roll over and die.

Now I am going to tell you some of the highlights of my health-kook journey. All of these things really happened.

A friend's mother got cancer on her face. It looked like a big wet oozing strawberry. I asked my friend what the doctor was going to do. The doctor, she told me, recommended doing nothing. Nothing? Nothing. His rationale was that my friend's mother was already pretty old. She had other, more pressing, health issues. So she might as well keep that cancer on her face.

"I wouldn't accept that if I were you," I said.

My friend didn't want to accept it either.

I gave her some homemade colloidal silver. This is tiny particles of silver, suspended in water.

"Wet a towel with this. Keep it damp, and keep it on the cancer."

The old lady liked watching TV, so she watched TV with a damp towel on her cheek. Whenever the towel got dry, she just dampened it again. After a week, the raw, red strawberry closed over with a scab. After two weeks, the scab got smaller. After three weeks…

"How's your mom's cancer?"

"Oh, it's gone. It fell off."

"It did what?"

"She went to wash her face in the morning, and it fell off. Fell into the sink."

"The scab?"

"Yes."

"And what was under the scab?"

"Just beautiful, healthy skin."

After this, my own parents-in-law's dog, Blackie, got cancer behind her left ear. Blackie was a gorgeous black Labrador Retriever. The cancer was a bloody raw sore, like my friend's mother's.

"What does the vet say?" I asked my wife.

"The vet says to watch and monitor."

"So you mean, to do nothing?"

"Yes."

I sighed, and gave my wife a spray bottle of good old homemade colloidal silver. "Tell your mom and dad to spray behind Blackie's ear as often as possible, I said. Keep it good and wet."

Two weeks later, my wife came home from visiting her parents. I asked how Blackie was doing, expecting good news.

"Not good, I'm afraid. The cancer's still there."

"Any change?"

"No change."

"But they are still spraying?"

"Actually, no, sorry."

What happened was this. They sprayed her cancer once. One time only. Blackie didn't like it, so they stopped.

The next Sunday we went to my in-law's. I brought a little bottle of colloidal silver. After lunch, I wetted a face towel. Blackie was lying on the floor. I lay down on top of her, adopting a wrestling hold. I won't lie: I was scared. A dog mauled me once, in my groin, and it wasn't much fun.

"Sorry, Blackie," I said. Then I gritted my teeth, grabbed her ear, and pressed the face towel into the bloody sore. Blackie cried in pain, but she let me do it. She squirmed, but didn't fight me.

"Please be careful, Hengist," said my parents-in-law, who didn't like this at all. But we stayed locked together on the floor, Blackie and me, until that face towel was dry.

Blackie got the face towel treatment once, only once, and her cancer went away. The sore dried up and turned into healthy skin. Healthy fur came back and covered it over.

My bank-manager friend told me, in conversation, that he was living with chronic pain. He had been in a car crash several years before, and had broken his back. Since that crash he had never enjoyed a moment free of pain.

"What, even now? Right now, as we sit here talking?"

"Yes, sure. Of course. Always."

"You hide it well."

"I've had a lot of practice," he shrugged.

I gave him a bottle of DMSO with a roll-on applicator.

"What's this?"

"Dimethyl sulfoxide," I said. "It's a molecule from trees. It's perfectly safe except it smells a bit like garlic and oysters, and it might make you itch. But if you put it on your back, I think your pain will go away. Just have your wife roll it on, after your bath."

"No thanks," he said, sliding it back across the table. "I don't believe in stuff like that."

"I do," I said, sliding it back. "Try it for me. What have you got to lose?"

My friend agreed he had nothing to lose. He also had nothing left to try. Bank managers, if you don't know, earn a pretty good living. My friend had money coming out of his ears. He had tried all the best doctors, and paid for all their children's private school tuitions.

After a week he returned the bottle. "You can have this back," he said. "It isn't working."

"Try a little longer," I told him. "The damage is deep, and it's been there for years. Might take a little longer to undo. Keep trying. Just for me."

I saw him two weeks later. He returned the bottle again, more insistently.

"You can have this back!"

I know when to give up, so I apologized.

"No, no. You don't understand. It worked. My pain is gone. You can have it back because I don't need it anymore. I'm all better!"

His chronic pain was gone. My friend joined a gym and got active again, something he used to love doing. This was several years ago, and the pain has never come back.

A friend's twin boys had acne. "Bad acne," she said.

"Show me," I said. She showed me a photo. It was a mess of blood and pus in 3D high-relief. Probably the worst acne I've ever seen.

"They're pretty depressed about it," she said, closing her phone on that horrible mess. "They're just getting ready to start high school. High school can be rough."

"Tell me about it," I shuddered. "Hang on. I have something that might help." I gave her twin spray bottles of a skin tonic I was making. The key ingredients were two botanicals and one mineral compound. "Have them spray their faces with this," I told my friend. "It will sting like the dickens, but tell them to embrace the pain, like men."

The mineral compound in my tonic is a halide salt. Spraying salt on gooey bloody acne was going to hurt, I knew. I was, at the time, using this same tonic as an aftershave. And I have always been a clumsy shaver. I knew the pain well.

"Tell them to see who's tougher. Make it a competition."

A few days later, my friend sent me fresh photos. There were her boys, beaming into the camera, not one pimple between them. Their faces were clear except for dark marks that were already fading.

For mild juvenile atopy, I hand out little spray bottles of colloidal silver. I tell the kids to carry a bottle in their pocket, or in their pencil case, and spray the areas as often as they can. The kids are always keen, but their parents are understandably wary.

"The doctor told us to keep the skin dry," they say.

"That's because the itchiness of atopy is caused by bacterial infection," I say. "Usually staphylococcal or streptococcal bacteria. Plain water encourages the bacterial growth. But this colloidal silver water will kill them. Splash it on, as much as you can. Also spray their bedsheets and pillows."

Mild atopy clears up fast. Severe atopy is harder, and the longer you've had it, the harder it is to get rid of. Most people just give up and try to live with it. Our pediatrician's adult son has severe atopy. She, a physician, and her husband, also a physician, had tried everything medical. She asked me what I would do.

"How bad is it, exactly?"

It was bad. Her son looked like a burn victim. He looked like a mummy.

"It will hurt like hell," I said. "But try this skin tonic. Also, try this colloidal silver. Tell him to use them in turns. I have no idea how much, how often, or what ratio. He'll have to be his own guinea pig. But as long as he wants to try, I'll keep supplying him."

It did hurt like hell, and he loved it. It helped him more than anything else he had tried. I gave his mom the recipe for the tonic, and showed her how her son could make his own colloidal silver.

"This is a miracle," she said. "I wish I could prescribe this to my patients."

"What do you mean?" I asked. "You can't? But you're the doctor. You can prescribe whatever you want."

Silly me. I was very naive.

My doctor friend had to explain that, no, a doctor is not free to prescribe just anything. The truth was the very opposite. They are strictly bound to a list of permitted drugs. They cannot deviate from this list. They cannot be creative. They cannot, as the saying goes, think outside the box.

"I'd be breaking the law," she said sadly. "I wish I could prescribe this, but I can't."

If there is an entrepreneur out there, a good businessman or woman, who wants to create a miraculous skin-care product that takes care of everything from pimples to severe atopy, and also stings like hell, please contact me. We'll be partners.

I was now buying an awful lot of spray bottles. I bought them by the case. I'd go to the shop, and say, "Two more cases of those cobalt-blue Boston-round spray bottles, please. One case of 50ml, and one of 100ml."

One day, I noticed that the shop manager was losing her hair.

"You're losing your hair," I said gently.

"Yes," she said. "Here." She pointed to a silver-dollar-sized bald spot, right in the front and center of her hairline.

"Do you work tomorrow? Yes? I will bring you back one of these bottles. Spray that bald spot as often as you think of it."

"Will it help?"

"I don't know."

The next time I went for a case of bottles, the shop manager ran at me as if she wanted to eat me, nom-nom-nom, like I was a big fat jelly donut. She was running and hopping and pointing with two hands at her head. The bald spot was gone. Her hairline was back.

I had a very dear friend who had the worst halitosis, like rotting meat. You knew when he entered the room. You smelled him coming a mile away.

It wasn't his fault, either. It wasn't a case of bad hygiene. My poor friend had tried everything from mouthwashes to gum surgery. Nothing helped. Bad breath like that is no joke. It hurt his quality of life. For one thing, it limited his employment opportunities. Also his love life. I made colloidal silver for him by the gallon. He swished and rinsed and gargled, and stuck with it till the stink went away. It took time, but it worked. He is happily married today, with children.

A friend's son broke his collarbone. You can't immobilize a broken collarbone. You can't wrap it in a plaster cast. The boy was in constant pain. What's worse, his soccer-playing was suspended. This boy loved soccer in a serious way. He was a budding star. The family had even designed their work and living arrangements around this boy's soccer-playing.

"Do you think your colloidal silver could help him?" she asked me.

"No."

"Oh."

"But there's something I've read about. Never used it. Only read about it. It's an herb. If you'd like to try it, I'll get some."

She was willing, so I ordered a bottle of comfrey oil. It arrived about one month into the broken bone. The boy had been ordered off the soccer field for at least three months.

My friend went home and rubbed this oil on her son. Ouch, ouch. Then she put him to bed. The next morning, he was looking cheerful. They put more oil on. Later that evening, when my friend came home from work, her son was waiting by the door.

"Look, mom! Look!" He was swinging his arm all around. She told him to stop. He would hurt himself! But he said it didn't hurt, and kept swinging it. "I can play soccer!"

She made him a deal. Keep your arm still, and keep putting on that oil. At the end of the week, we'll see the doctor.

The boy's doctor couldn't deny that swinging, windmilling arm. He ordered an x-ray. The x-ray showed that the bone had healed unnaturally fast.

"The boy may play soccer," he ruled. "Just go a little easy, and don't fall down."

Comfrey also goes by the names knitbone and boneset. It's a wonderful herb, and since my wife and I have had children, we try to keep a bottle always handy.

This next story looks a little like witchcraft, but it is true. A friend of mine suddenly started crying. I asked her what was wrong. She had been to the doctor earlier that day, because of headaches. The doctor ordered scans, and found a brain aneurysm. An artery was bulging, and threatening to pop. It was like a time-bomb. In her brain. I knew nothing about aneurysms, but after all, we do have the internet, don't we. First I had to crack the spelling. That done, I read a few things. The next time I saw my friend, I gave her some supplements and a copper kettle.

"All of the water that you use, for drinking or cooking, you are going to boil in this kettle," I told her. "Coffee, tea, soup, eggs, potatoes, spaghetti, whatever. All the water gets boiled in this. Do you understand?"

She understood. The poor girl took my supplements and my kettle. At her next couple of monitoring appointments, the aneurysm was still there. And then, at around her third or fourth visit, it wasn't there. It had "resolved." The girl's brain was no longer in danger of exploding. She got on with life, became married, and has two children now.

Why the kettle? I had read that aneurysms can be caused by copper deficiency. So I gave her the copper kettle. Later, I thought, "Duh, Earth to Hengist Mountebank. She couldn't have got much copper from your kettle. That copper kettle was lined with tin!" Witchcraft or not, her aneurysm did go away.

A friend of mine revealed to me one day that she had an invalid son. I say we were friends, and we were friendly. I had known her, by this time, for about two years. But she never spoke to me about her family. And I never asked. I didn't even know that she had children. I knew about her husband, that he was very wealthy - important to this story. Anyway, I asked her what was wrong.

Her son was about my age. He was married. Had three children. Was healthy, to all appearances. But - it turned out - he had a time-bomb in his brain, and it exploded. One day he was at work, working, and then he fell down from a massive stroke.

"When?"

"Three years ago."

"And how is he now?"

"He's still in the hospital. The doctors say he'll never walk or talk again."

"Good heavens!"

"It's okay. He's comfortable. We're used to it now."

Some people have an amazing ability to resign themselves to things. I admire this attitude sometimes. But sometimes not. I started looking into strokes.

I didn't have to look far. In Dr. Walker's book I found a study done in Argentina and Chile on geriatric stroke victims. DMSO was given both orally and intramuscularly. After the treatment period, doctors assessed the patients' therapeutic results. Seventy-four percent (74.35) found themselves in the Good category. Nearly twenty-two percent (21.77) were in the Fair category. Under four percent (3.88) received a score of Zero. This looked very hopeful, so I took it to my friend.

"It's interesting," she said. "But I don't think the doctors will allow it."

"With respect, it's not the doctor's decision. They don't even have to know."

"I suppose not," she said. "But my husband! My husband would never allow it."

"With the greatest of respect, it isn't his decision, either. It's your son's. You don't necessarily have to tell your husband, either."

Her look told me I was walking on thin ice. Thin, cracking ice. I might lose a friend if I pushed this. But her son, and his family, were depending on me to push it. Who else knew about this South American study? Who else was looking? Not the doctors. They'd said three years ago there's nothing they could do for the man. They'd quit trying. They'd resigned him, as his own mother had done, to his miserable, crippled, mute existence.

"I think you should ask your son," I said. "Give him this information. Ask him what he would like to do. Can he communicate?"

He could grunt. He could blink yes or no.

"Good. So go, have a talk with your son."

The next time I saw her, she was excited.

"He wants to do it!"

The South American study described a complicated protocol involving injections and ampoules, neither of which we had. So I told my friend, just smuggle it in in your purse, and put it in his orange juice. How much? I don't know. Let's try one ounce of DMSO at breakfast, lunch, and dinner.

We waited.

The son slowly improved. By days and by weeks. The more DMSO in orange juice he drank, the better he got. The use of his limbs returned. He started speaking again. Then he got into a wheelchair. Then he got out of the wheelchair, and onto crutches. After about a year, he was out of the hospital.

Today he plays with his children again. He cooks for his family. He works. He walks 2 km to work, works at his job, and walks home. "I could drive," he says. "Or I could bicycle. But I know what it's like not to be able to walk. So I like to walk. I really, really like to walk."

Well, I could go on. But that is my health-kook career in a nutshell. You can see how it just kind of snowballed from my father-in-law's cancer diagnosis until I was going around town healing pimples and baldness and broken backs and everything else.

Oh, and I should tell you how it went for my father-in-law. He played out his bad odds and beat them. He smashed through his 7% five-year survival. He crashed through 10 years like a legend. The last 1 or 2 years were hard. But he got about 10 really good and happy years. He worked on his farm, which he loved. He outlived Blackie, and got another Black Lab, and called that one Blackie, too. He got to see, at last, our first daughter, Matilda. His first grandchild, and the only one he got to see. He didn't get to meet Florentina. But he loved our Matilda. And she loved him. They were great together.

As he lay dying, we all stood around his bed. Matilda was in my arms. Father-in-law gazed and gazed at her. He knew he had not much time left. All he wanted, it seemed, was to drink her in with his eyes. If anyone spoke to him, he acknowledged them. But his eyes kept coming back and resting on Matilda.

Father-in-law loved me. He treated me like his own son. He taught me much. The biggest thing he taught me - he taught me by the way he looked at Matilda that day. Everyday, everyday, I try to see my daughters with his eyes.

Father-in-law, from where you are now, I hope you can see them through mine.

2
INFERTILITY

I like knives. I have knives for the kitchen, knives for my pants pockets, knives for the garden, and knives for the bush. I have knives I will never use because they are too beautiful. I don't want to get them dirty. I'm not a real collector or anything. I don't know anything about knives. I don't read knife magazines. Thinking about it now, I can only think of two maker's names. I just like knives. I don't know. I think they're cool.

The best knife shop in town is just a 5-minute walk from my office. I used to go there just to look at the beautiful, beautiful knives. Sometimes I would go home with an impulse buy. Another paring knife, or sushi knife, or meat-cleaver, or bone-handled field dressing blade, or axe.

I promoted that shop to everybody, too. "If you need a knife, go to Mr Cutler's shop," I'd say. "He's a real nice old guy, and he has the best knives." Well, this is a gossipy little town, and one day someone hit me with some gossip about Mr Cutler.

"Did you know that this is his second marriage?"

"No." I didn't know. Nor did I care.

"Oh, let me tell you! He was married before! When he was younger!"

"Oh?" I wasn't interested. I was trying to be a polite listener. But now I wish I had said, *Excuse me, I don't care about the man's past. It's none of my beeswax, or yours.*

"Yes," said my friend. "His first wife wasn't able to have a baby, so he divorced her and remarried."

I kept my composure. "Oh," I said. "That's very sad." But I felt as if my friend had taken one of Mr Cutler's knives and stabbed me right in the heart. I wanted to punch my gossipy friend right in her stupid gossipy teeth.

My wife and I were 5 or 6 years into marriage at the time, and 5 or 6 years into infertility. Well, on the bright side, looking back now, we were about halfway through! But of course we didn't know that at the time. Childlessness, barrenness, lifelessness, unfruitfulness, sterility, infertility, or whatever you call it looked like those deserts in Lawrence of Arabia: lifeless, endless, and hopeless. Or like a cartoon bottomless pit. You keep falling and falling and falling, without even the resolution of a splat.

If I ever need another knife, I will still go back to Mr Cutler's. He does have the best knife shop in town. But the truth is, I already have an awful lot of knives. Probably I have enough to last me a lifetime. Once in a while I do go back there, just to visit and say hello. But not so often. It isn't that I judge Mr Cutler. It just feels awkward.

Maybe it's for the best. Maybe the first Mrs Cutler was a really horrible person. Maybe she had a violent temper and lacked every maternal instinct. Maybe she would have been the kind of parent who leaves their children in hot parked cars. Maybe it's best that she never came anywhere near a child. But let's face it, she was probably a perfectly nice person.

I mentioned earlier that a junkyard dog once mauled me in my groin. My wife and I were dating at the time, and engaged to be married. As a matter of fact we were together on a date when this crazed dog attacked me. (Not without reason. Its collar was digging into its neck, cutting through the flesh. I was trying to loosen the collar. The dog did not know that. It reacted like any semi-feral, threatened animal in pain.)

CHOMP.

One jaw dug into my hand, and one jaw dug into my thigh, just around my groin. It was a rainy day, fortunately. My wife had her umbrella. We were able, with the tip of it, to pry the dog's jaws loose, and I slipped free.

I was damned lucky that he didn't get my femoral artery. I might have bled out. Also, as Dr. T. tells me, damned lucky that I didn't develop sepsis, leading to amputation or death. At the time, though, my focus was rather narrower.

"Damned lucky he didn't get the old meat and taters!" I said to my bride to be.

Yes, she agreed.

A foolish idea came into my head. I, being a fool, gave it voice.

"Say, I think there's a Hemingway story about a guy who gets shot in the groin, or gored by a bull. And he loves the girl, but he gives her up because he was shot or gored in the groin. Hey, if that darned dog really did get my meat and 'taters, you would still marry me, right?"

My wife is no fool. Nor does she suffer them gladly. Her tongue poked her cheek as she thought about it for about two and a half seconds.

"No," she said. "No, I wouldn't. I'm marrying you because I want to have a family with you."

For the first time in my life, I felt like a sex object. But soon we would get married and find out that we were infertile. Feeling like a sex object - a *broken* sex object - got to be very familiar.

We were lucky in this: the doctors didn't know who was defective, my wife or me. Or maybe they knew and didn't tell us. If so, they did the right thing. My wife and I could have ended up like Mr. Cutler's first marriage. Better not to know, better not to know. That way we could each doubt *ourselves*, and loathe *ourselves*. My wife felt for certain it was her fault. I felt for certain it was mine.

You might be in the same situation. You may not know where the problem is. Or you may think you know. Or you may know you know. It doesn't matter! It really doesn't. When I was a boy, I used to take piping hot baths. My dad always told me I'd make myself sterile. I didn't listen. I liked my bath water hot!

Whether my dad was truly concerned about my reproductive future, or whether he was primarily concerned with his heating bill, the point is this: lost and dying in the desert of infertility, I blamed those hot baths. I blamed myself for boiling my balls to death.

Furthermore, I'd taken quite a few punches to the nuts, in my time. A few knees. And a few soccer balls, and one or two baseballs. I used to daredevil my bike off a cliff into the creek, and come down hard on my banana-seat. Once or twice I sat down on my nuts and squashed them.

My wife, meanwhile, blamed herself. She had, or invented, her own reasons. Whatever. It didn't matter in the end.

Whatever the doctors are telling you, or whatever you are suspecting, it doesn't matter yet - unless it makes you give up. The doctors know what they know. That's fine. They don't know about DMSO. They don't know what it did for my wife and me. Have hope! And I know that this is the hardest thing for you, now. To have hope.

How many times did I come home in the evening to find my wife with puffy face and puffy eyes. "Good news," she would tell me, lip quivering.

Oh boy. My heart would rip a little more, and I would take her in my arms, and hear her news. Another friend had gotten pregnant. Another friend had had a baby.

We loved our friends. We were happy for them. And it also, to us, always felt like a cosmic "fuck-you." Sorry for the bad language, but that is the best way to describe it. It felt like the Lord God, you know, on the roof of the Sistine Chapel there, was stretching out his arm to raise a big old middle finger in our faces.

Still hoping for that baby? Still praying to me? You know what? FUCK YOU.

Not proud of it. We both feel ashamed of it, now and then. I know you do, too. It is undoubtedly wrong and sinful to feel that way. But it's also perfectly human and natural. When Abraham's wife, Sarah, doubted God, she was doubting God's overt promise. You and I never had a promise from God to rest on. It is very much harder for us to keep the faith. And yet, we must keep it.

Meanwhile, friends get pregnant; friends have babies. People get pregnant by accident. People abort their babies. People have babies in toilets, and leave them there. People toss their babies into dumpsters. People abuse their babies. People rape their babies. People neglect their babies. You and I, we somehow have to keep faithful throughout all this!

It's like this. My wife and I got married in a church. Hopeful scriptures were read over us. Prayers were sent up for us. "Be fruitful and multiply," we thought was the plan. We believed that was the plan!

Every month, we hoped our first baby would arrive. The first of many. We'd wait, as people wait for loved ones in airport arrivals. Big expectant grins on faces. Big homemade signs, saying WELCOME BABY.

Those arrival doors slide open and close, and babies come out. You stand on tiptoes to see. Is that one mine? Is that one? Maybe that one? The next one, surely? Pretty soon now, honey! They're thinning out now! Can't be long now!

All the babies are received into loving or unloving arms and driven away. It's just you two now, all alone, staring at an empty luggage carousel. *Clack-clack, clack-clack, clack-clack.* Honey, you have to move. The janitor wants to mop there.

The first dozen or two-dozen times you feel like an idiot. You feel like you must have gone to the wrong airport. You screwed up the date, or the flight number. Anyway, it's your fault.

Let me tell you, after four-dozen or six-dozen times, you begin to realize, no, we're doing everything right. We're not stupid. It's not our fault.

We are being cruelly pranked.

The temptation, then, is to rip up your WELCOME BABY sign, and shove it in the garbage. And then drive home, and tear down all the welcome decorations, and out of spite maybe light the whole house on fire.

We made that trip not six-dozen times, not eight-dozen times, but ten-dozen times! And we frequently did rip up our signs and decorations. We stopped short of lighting the house on fire, but we did out of spite and despair and weariness stop trying, and stop praying. We said things we shouldn't.

"We'll never have a baby."

"It's hopeless."

"There's nothing left to try."

"We don't need a baby."

"We can be happy without a baby."

"I don't even want a baby, anymore."

"I don't even want to be married, anymore."

Always, in the end, we'd go and pick our ripped signs and decorations out of the trash, and meekly tape them back together.

Other couples did give up. Some, probably too early. They stoically resigned themselves, like my friend stoically resigned her stroke-stricken son to his sickbed, to be a mute cripple for life. She resigned him too soon!

Oh, Reader. Perhaps the doctor told you that you have about a 1% chance of ever getting pregnant. You feel that's pretty measly, and it is. But it's still infinitely better than a zero percent chance. And I guess the doctor didn't tell you that you have a zero percent chance, or you probably wouldn't have bothered to read this book!

But let's say that your doctor has told you that your chances are flat out zero. Unless you are missing major parts of your body because of a catastrophic dog-mauling or bull-goring, I would fire that doctor and find a decent one. Because you just never know for sure. And your dumb doctor sure doesn't know for sure, either.

Based on all of our evidence and experience, my wife and I had a zero percent chance of having a baby. After about 120 months? Get out of here. Do the math. We were about as hopeless a case as there's ever been.

That's why I don't care very much about your physical condition. Or what the doctor has told you. The physical struggle is secondary. If you give up mentally, or emotionally, or spiritually, then the physical challenge is lost by forfeit.

Don't give up.

I know, I know. Sex isn't fun anymore. It feels not even loving anymore. It feels like work. Like a dreaded household chore. Worse than a chore! You can do your chores and have the satisfaction that they're done. The house is tidied. The laundry is folded. The toilets are clean. But with this, it's like mopping a dirty floor with a dirty mop. It's getting nowhere! You feel like a robot in a factory - a factory that produces nothing.

Making it worse, there are strangers involved. "Sex is between two married people who love each other." Is that what your mother told you? How quaint. No, sex is between you and your doctors and nurses and technicians, thank you very much. It used to be private and personal. Now you have these guys sticking in their noses and gloved hands...

BEEP. Oh, the thermometer says you're supposed to get aroused now. You know what I mean. Pretend to get aroused. Pretend to be interested. Pretend to be into it. Draw on old memories. You used to be into this. You used to climax together...

Now, only one of you needs to climax, and that sadly, into a test tube.

You might be feeling that you're at the lowest point in your life, your miserable life. I respect that. You might not want to be encouraged. I respect that. You might hate all the idiots who tell you to keep on hoping, keep trying, keep praying. I respect that.

But buddy, you have to keep going. You just have to. Follow me, or don't follow me, but you have to keep going. You cannot just sit down here in no-man's land and give up. You just can't.

Because of the efforts and costs and indignities you're going through, whenever you finally do succeed, you will make better parents. You will make the *best* parents. Your children will be the most loved children. Your joys will be more joyful.

From *Heart with No Companion* by Leonard Cohen:

Now I greet you from the other side of sorrow and despair,

With a love so vast and shattered, it will reach you everywhere.

And I sing this for the captain whose ship has not been built,

For the mother in confusion, her cradle still unfilled.

For the heart with no companion, for the soul without a king.

For the prima ballerina who cannot dance to anything.

This is me, greeting you from the other side, you mothers and fathers in confusion. Your cradles still unfilled. Greeting you with love, and encouragement, and if necessary a boot up your backside. You have to keep going! Up! Up! And onward! And if you think there are already too many mixed metaphors here, now I am strapping into my A-10 Warthog, and flying ahead of you, straight into the face of our common enemy! *Brrrrrrrrrrrrrrrrrrrrrrrrrrrrrrrrrrrrrrrrrrrrrrrrrrrrrraaaaaaaaaaaaaaaaap!*

3
EUREKA!

*I*t's a funny old world. If my father-in-law hadn't gone and gotten cancer, I would never have travelled down Mountebank Lane, and our daughters would never have entered this life. It is almost as if my father-in-law sacrificed himself for their, and our, sakes.

Now here's the crazy thing. All of the time that I was wracking my brain over my father-in-law's cancer, and friends' and acquaintances ailments from bald spots and broken backs to aneurysms and hemorrhagic strokes, I never thought about studying infertility. I never thought of it! None of my herbs and pills and chemicals, and none of my other snake oils and contraptions, none of it, ever spoke to my wife and me. Why not? I don't know.

Maybe it's because I didn't see infertility as a medical kind of condition. I didn't see it as a disease. I saw it as personal failure and inadequacy and lack of manhood. This was a wrong and bad perspective, and a near fatal blindness. It almost cost my wife and me our children. I thank God, and give him the credit, for snapping me out of it.

Okay now, this is what did it. I was reading about good old DMSO, my trusty molecule from trees. Oh, the many adventures that we had gone through together, my good old sidekick DMSO and me.

I was just picking my nose one day, and reading about DMSO, and I came across something that I had never read before. No, that' can't be true. I had surely read it before and never appreciated it because I was a massive dummy.

DMSO, dimethyl sulfoxide, is employed in the storage and transportation of organs, for the purpose of organ transplantation.

[*A bolt of lightning strikes my head. Explodes my brain.*]

4
EUREKA EXPLAINED FOR MASSIVE DUMMIES LIKE ME

*G*ather around my feet now, all you little dummies, and let your Uncle Dum-dum spell this eureka moment out for you. I will teach you by way of a parable.

One fine day, on one side of the country, a young man is speeding down the freeway on his motorcycle. His name is Chad, and he is a cad. A bad cad named Chad. Look at him go, boys and girls. See his luxurious mullet streaming behind him, as he weaves in and out of traffic. He is endangering himself and other motorists. What can be his hurry? Where is he going so fast? He is going to rendezvous with a woman of low character, and to cheat on his lovely but frustratingly imperceptive girlfriend, whose name is Betty Trueheart.

Meanwhile, over on the other side of the country, Betty's very double (played by the same actress) is clinging to life, but just. This doppelgänger's name? By fantastic coincidence, her name is *Bessie Trueheart*.

"Bessie has mere hours now," her doctor tells her parents. "She may not live the night."

"Can nothing else be done?"

The doctor shakes his head. "No. Her little heart is giving up. It is too tired. There remains only to pray for a miracle."

Meanwhile, back over on Chad's side of the country, a trucker named Bud "The Spud" Spudman is hauling a 20-ton load of potatoes. Suddenly - a miracle! Bud's coffee falls out of his hand and into his lap. Scalding hot! Fumbling with both hands! The colossal 18-wheeler swerves erratically...

A short time later, at the hospital.

"Yep, that's him." Chad's mom identifies her son. "That's my Chad. Is he dead?"

"He *is* still alive in a technical sense," says the doctor. "But in a totally vegetative state." He speaks in a clipped manner because he is going to be late for dinner.

"What does that mean?"

"It means that his brain is as unresponsive as a vegetable," says the blunt medical man, casting a furtive glance at his wristwatch. "As unresponsive as that truckload of potatoes that toppled over and crushed him. As unresponsive as the broccoli I had at lunch."

"But he will get better?"

"No. He will never get better. There is no hope of that. When I said that his brain is like potatoes and broccoli, I want you to understand that it is like *mashed* potatoes, and *overcooked, grey-green, falling apart, hospital-cafeteria* broccoli."

"Oh dear."

"So I would like to unplug these machines, and free up this bed, and let your son go to his well-earned rest."

Chad's mom fidgets a space.

"Yeah, I guess so," she says.

"Good. Just one more thing. The rest of him, from his brain on down, is all fine. We'd like to use him for spare parts, if you don't mind."

"Sure, why not," Chad's mom agrees. She just wants to get out of here. Get out of this place of sickness and death. Get out of this place of horror. Get out of this place of no-smoking.

"Good, thank you," says the doctor, winking to the nurse to take over. "You'll have to sign a few forms. Brenda, here, will help you. Very sorry for your loss. Goodbye."

Within the hour, the organ harvesting team has descended on Chad like a flock of vultures on a Zoroastrian *dakhma*, those "towers of silence" constructed for the singular grim purpose of excarnation.

"Eyeballs," says the eyeball man, a distinguished old surgeon holding what looks, to the untrained eye, like an ordinary household grapefruit spoon.

"Here," says the eyeball nurse. She holds a little cooler box for eyeballs. *Plop, plop.* The eyeball man plops the eyeballs in.

"Spleen," says the spleen man.

"Here," says the spleen nurse, with the spleen cooler. *Plop*.

"Appendix," says the appendix man.

"Here," says the appendix nurse. *Plop*.

"Big toe," says the big toe man.

"Big toe here." *Plop*.

"Mullet."

"Mullet." *Plop*.

"Heart," says the heart man.

"Heart, check." says the heart nurse. *Splash*. The hollow muscular organ splashes into the cooler box with a name and address written on its side. Whose name? And whose address? You have guessed it. The name is Bessie Twoheart, and the address is the address of the hospital where she lays languishing on her ostensible deathbed. For Chad's heart, you see, is going to *her*.

Now then, class of dummies. Is it becoming clear to you? These organs are going great distances. They might go across the whole country. That takes time. And do you know what organs, removed from the body, start to do? Immediately? That's right. They immediately start to decompose.

Then you are going to have ambulances hurrying these organs from airport to hospital. That takes time. Then you have to rush the organs from the parking lot to the operating room. You have swinging and sliding doors. Those take time. You have elevators. Those take time. Then I suppose you start opening up the recipient. That takes time. All of this takes time. From coast to coast, from Chad to Bessie, it's going to be several hours. Have you ever left a steak out on your counter for just one hour? Have you seen the changes that start going on after just one hour?

Okay, let's play a guessing game. When they packed those cooler boxes, and you heard the plops and splashes, what else do you think they put in there? I mean, besides the organs. They don't just dump the organs in an empty box, to bang around and get all bruised. What do they use to protect them?

Styrofoam peanuts? No.

Old newspaper? No.

Oily rags? No.

Ice cubes from the local convenience store? No.

Saline solution? No.

Blood? No.

Plasma? No.

Formaldehyde? No.

Pickle juice? No.

Coconut milk? Good guess, but no.

I can see you're not even enjoying this game, so I will just tell you.

They put the organs in DMSO.

[*Dramatic Chipmunk theme, moderate volume.*]

5

FOR THE TRULY AND HOPELESSLY DENSE

Some of you have made the connection. Others have not. So let's examine a general problem, and then see if that sheds any light on a specific problem.

General problem: How to transport organs or cells from one place to another, and from one body to another, in tiptop condition? Answer: DMSO.

Specific problem: How to transport sperm cells from my testicles to my wife's womb, also in tiptop condition? Answer:

[*Dramatic Chipmunk theme, extra loud.*]

Very good. DMSO. That is the same conclusion that I came to. For it seemed to me very reasonable that if DMSO can carry a heart 3,000 miles across a continent, from donor to recipient, then it ought to be able to carry my sperm the short distance from my testicles to my wife's egg. If it can keep a heart fresh and lively for hours, then it ought to keep my sperm fresh and lively for what a few minutes? Oh, here. The internet tells me a fast-swimming sperm can make it to the egg in thirty minutes. Perfect!

This was my Big Idea. This was my lightning bolt. The apple falling on my head. No. This was the whole apple *tree* falling on my head. The moment it connected in my brain, I knew it would work. I didn't know why it would work. I just knew it was going to work!

More research only confirmed me in my belief. Spermatozoa and ova are routinely preserved, even frozen, in DMSO solutions. It is the routine way of preserving sperm and eggs. Why not employ this marvellous substance in the treatment of infertility? It seemed too obvious. Someone in the fertility world should have thought of it by now.

Doubt crept in.

I'm being too simple, I thought. Some things are too good to be true. DMSO? It's too easy. And most of all, it's too cheap. From experience I knew that fertility treatments have to be expensive! Because fertility treatments *are* expensive, right? Then I thought about it more, from the money angle.

Sure, fertility treatments are expensive. But they can't be expensive compared with a heart transplant operation. I search-engined that. An average heart transplant costs about $1,500,000.

Okay. Let's suspend all humanity, and concentrate on that money. Who pays it? I don't know, but I imagine it has got to be insurance companies. Or at least it would have to go through insurance companies and be approved by them. Are insurance companies notoriously profligate with money? No. Are they notoriously kooky and sloppy? Are they *mountebanks*?

No, of course not. Insurance companies are notoriously smart and cautious and greedy.

So let's trust that the insurance companies are not carelessly throwing their money away, as my wife and I threw our money away on those white-teethed fertility doctors and their country clubs and sports cars. Insurance companies don't throw money away.

If you're an insurance company, and you're holding the risk on a million-dollar heart transplantation, do you think you're doing everything you can to reduce that risk? You bet you are. You think you're doing your homework? You're darn right you are. You're studying the subject, you're consulting all the experts, and you're taking care of every smallest detail. Like, you'll probably have a guy at the recipient's hospital at such-and-such a time, holding the elevator door open. Little details like that.

When you're deciding what is the best possible substance for keeping the heart in the best possible condition, that is not a small detail. That is a hugely important detail. If the insurance companies and hospital boards are all going with DMSO, then I figure I'm pretty safe going with DMSO. Follow the money. The big money bets on DMSO.

Doubt crept out.

Okay then. The shape of a plan was settling out in my mind.

Use DMSO to prep my sperm, make it all vigorous and dynamic, and transport it from A (me) to B (my wife, or namely, her egg). Good enough for a million-dollar transplantation operation, good enough for us. That was settled in my mind. How to do it? Getting the DMSO inside my scrotum, and inside my testicles, that was going to be the easy part. That would pose no difficulty at all.

The hard part, and the crucial part, would be getting my sperm inside my wife without her knowledge. For this was going to be a Top Secret operation.

You may frown on me for this. I know there are ethical questions involved. Informed consent, and so on. But no, I couldn't tell her. Here's why. We'd been going at this thing for 10 years. We had had approximately 120 months of dashed hopes. Our hopes were smashed about as flat as Chad when a truckload of potatoes fell on him. Our marriage, too, was feeling kind of flat. My wife and my marriage couldn't take much more disappointment. I couldn't raise her hopes. I wouldn't do it. That was my firm feeling.

So here was my mission.

Get DMSO inside my testicles. The more, the better!

Get my turbo-assisted power-sperm inside my wife, at precisely the right moment, without her knowing!

6
SCIENCE STUFF

This and the next chapter will be a bit dry. We are going to look in this chapter at the science of DMSO, and in the following chapter at safety. Then I will return to me and my cunning plan to impregnate my wife without her knowledge.

Dimethyl sulfoxide (DMSO) is an organosulfur compound. It is an elegant little molecule with neat symmetry. Its head is an oxygen atom. Its body is a sulfur atom. And then it has two limbs, each composed of three carbon atoms bonded to one hydrogen atom. All very neat and proper. I have seen the molecule illustrated in both skinny and fat versions. The skinny version looks a little like the Road Runner. The fat version looks a lot like the Michelin Man.

As you have already learned, this molecule is made inside trees. It comes out of them as a byproduct of the pulp and paper industry. Pulp mill workers are among those who discovered some of its uses. Handling DMSO, they found, made the older guys' arthritis go away. It also worked great for cleaning the chrome on their cars.

Russian scientist Alexander Saytzeff first synthesized DMSO in 1866. He described it as a colorless liquid, similar to a mineral oil, having an oily texture, a garlicky odor, and an aftertaste reminiscent of clams or oysters. Saytzeff also found it to be an excellent solvent, degreaser, paint thinner, and antifreeze. For most of the next 100 years, DMSO performed mostly in industrial capacities. Please do not let these words make you nervous. Water is the universal solvent. Olive oil, that's another super scary solvent. Lemon juice is an excellent degreaser. Vinegar, too. Turpentine is a paint thinner, and it's also found in most chest rubs and inhalers. The gin in my freezer is an antifreeze.

In 1959, DMSO broke into the medical field. British scientists showed that it protected red blood cells and other tissues in freezing conditions. From this, DMSO found its role as protector of organs in organ-transplants (our cooler boxes). Since 1962, DMSO has been used in the freezing of organs for long-term storage. DMSO is also used, currently, in cryonics: the freezing and (it is hoped) eventual unfreezing of billionaires who are afraid to meet their Maker.

DMSO has an uncanny ability to penetrate and pass through living tissues. I can show you this dramatically. Take off one shoe and one sock. Put your foot up on this ottoman. Here, I will paint a dab on the bottom of your foot. Twenty seconds later, you will taste it in your mouth, inside your very tongue! Because that's where it is, in the blood vessels of your tongue. That's how powerfully and quickly it entered your bloodstream. From your foot.

This property is exploited in medicine, where DMSO is used to carry drugs inside the body. For DMSO is also an excellent solvent, remember. Dissolve an antibiotic, or an anesthetic, or an anti-cancer drug in DMSO, and paint it on the body. The DMSO will carry the drug where needles cannot go. Brain tumor? DMSO can pass the blood-brain barrier. In a few minutes DMSO can go right through your skull.

DMSO has the rather bizarre property of loving water, and being attracted to water, even more than water is attracted to itself. The bond of DMSO to water is 1.3 times as strong as the bond of water to water. Because of this it gets deeply into tissues, and deeply into cells, making itself quite at home, displacing and replacing some of the water that is in there. Dr. Walker goes into this more, in his book. He feels that this water attraction *"probably is what makes DMSO an entirely different healing power than anything medical science has known before."* (His italics.)

DMSO is therefore diuretic and drying. If you use it topically, you will find that it has a drying-out effect on your skin. This is useful in the healing of burns, where moisture promotes infection. Also in the treatment of inflammation and swelling, including swelling of the brain. I have found DMSO to be very good for a stuffy or dripping nose. Paint two fingertips with DMSO. Insert into nostrils. Give a few good turns. Remove fingers. You will be able to breathe easily

This versatile molecule stimulates production of white blood cells, and of the migration inhibitory factor (MIF) of macrophages. MIF has been described as the body's ever-present natural chemotherapy against cancer.

DMSO is, by itself, antibacterial, antiviral, antifungal, and anti-cancerous.

DMSO is used both in mainstream and alternative cancer treatments, both with other substances (e.g. DMSO-hematoxylon, or DMSO-cesium chloride) and alone. At Mount Sinai Hospital, New York City, Dr. Charlotte Friend has turned cancerous cells back into normal healthy ones by putting them into test tubes with DMSO solutions.

As you have read, DMSO is used to carry anesthetics into the body. But DMSO is, itself, a powerful anesthetic, by blocking conduction in the small c-fibers, the unsheathed or nonmyelinated nerve fibers.

A remarkable anecdote to demonstrate the pain-killing power of DMSO, if you don't mind. Dr. William Campbell Douglass practiced medicine in Saratoga, Florida. One day, a little six-year-old girl named Penelope stuck her finger into a live light socket. Her finger must have gotten stuck because it was in the socket for some period of time. Her index finger was "cooked through and burned ash white at the tip." Within 30 minutes, Dr. Douglass had the screaming child's finger soaking in full-strength DMSO. After 20 minutes of this, the girl had stopped crying. She felt no more discomfort. She slept well that night, and the next morning woke up with pink and healing finger. From the severity of her injury, it was thought that she would probably lose the finger, or at least its tip, from gangrene. Little Penelope instead made a complete and total recovery.

DMSO is an enthusiastic scavenger of free radicals, especially the hydroxyl free radicals, those little black-masked, bomb-toting anarchists that infiltrate human cells and blow them up. DMSO scoops up those free radicals, and sends them out in the urine.

Allergic reactions are suppressed or lessened by DMSO.

Look, we are hurrying along because I am not setting out to write a whole book on the marvellous properties and functions and applications of DMSO. Such books already exist. I am leaning heavily on one: DMSO Nature's Healer, by Dr. Morton Walker. I recommend it as the best place to start.

The literature on DMSO is vast. As of today, a search for "dimethyl sulfoxide" on PubMed, that wonderful tool of the US National Library of Medicine, National Institutes of Health, and the National Center for Biotechnology Information, returns 21,603 results for articles and studies. That number is always increasing. A search for "DMSO" returns 30,629 results.

Let's have a quick list of what DMSO does, and then let's have a quick list of conditions that DMSO has been used for.

DMSO does these things. It penetrates tissues and cells. It replaces water in tissues and cells. It stimulates immunity. It is anesthetic. It is anti-inflammatory. It is bacteriostatic, virostatic, and fungistatic. It acts against cancer. It carries drugs through membranes. It reduces platelet thrombi in blood vessels. It inhibits calcium, reducing the workload on the heart. It is a vasodilator, also reducing the workload on the heart. It is a tranquilizer. It softens and reduces collagen in the skin. It scavenges free radicals, especially hydroxyls. It is a potent diuretic. It is a reagent, speeding up chemical processes by as much as "a billionfold." It protects tissues and cells from freezing. It protects tissues and cells against radiation. It flushes toxins from tissues and cells. It suppresses allergic reactions. It dilates blood vessels. It improves circulation. And I have no doubt that it does many more things, both known and yet unknown.

Again, here is a non-exhaustive alphabetic list of ailments and conditions that DMSO has been used to treat. Have fun with your imagination by using what you have learned about DMSO's properties. Guess how it might be helping each illness.

Acne. Adenocarcinoma. AIDS. Alzheimer's. Amyloidosis. Ankle sprain. Arthritis. Asthma. Atherosclerosis. Athlete's foot. Athletic injuries. Back pain. Bile duct stones. Bladder inflammation. Bone cancer. Brain embolism. Brain trauma and stroke. Breast cancer. Bronchiolitis. Bruises. Bunions. Burns. Bursitis. Calluses. Cancer, generally. Carpal Tunnel syndrome. Cataracts. Cervical cancer. Cervical os, the stenosis of. Chemotherapy side-effects. Cirrhosis of the liver. Clubnails. Colon cancer. Corneal swelling. Corns. CREST syndrome. Cystic mastitis. Dancer's foot. Dandruff. Diabetes. Digestive problems. Down's syndrome. Dry socket. Ear infections. Facial cancer. Fallen arches. Fibromyalgia. Fibrosarcoma. Foot odor. Fractures. Fungus toenails. Gastrointestinal cancer. Glaucoma. Gout. Granulomatosis. Hammertoes. Head and spinal cord injuries. Headache. Hearing problems. Heart attacks. Heel spurs. Herpes simplex. Herpes zoster. Hives. Ingrown toenails. Intracranial hypertension. Keloids. Kidney cancer. Leiomyosarcoma. Leprosy. Leukopenia. Liver cancer. Lumbar disc problems. Lung cancer. Lung infections. Lupus. Lymphosarcoma. Macular degeneration. Macular edema. Melanoma. Metatarsalgia. Multiple sclerosis. Myasthenia gravis. Neurological disorders. Orchitis. Osteoarthritis. Osteomyelitis. Parasitic worms. Parenchymatous parotitis. Parkinsonism. Periodontal disease. Peyronie's disease. Phantom limb pain. Plantar warts. Respiratory infections. Retinitis pigmentosa. Reye's syndrome. Scars. Scleroderma. Senility. Sinusitis. Skin cancer. Still's disease. Stroke. Tendinitis. Tennis elbow. Tic douloureaux. Traumatic uveitis. Tubal obstruction. Ulcerations. Urinary system problems. Varicose veins.

And may I add to the list, in at least my family's case, Infertility.

I began with the simple thought that what is good for a million-dollar organ ought to be good for a single sperm cell. I guessed that the DMSO was sort of fluffing up the sperm, optimizing its health and protecting it somehow. I still think this. But now I think a second thing may have been going on. This is only a guess, of course.

I think that the DMSO, once inside my testicles, immediately started scavenging free radicals, especially the hydroxyl type. There is a large literature on hydroxyl radicals and male fertility/infertility rates, with titles like, *"Correlation Between Human Semen Mg and Hydroxyl Radical Levels and Human Spermiogram."* The news from these articles is bad. Hydroxyl free radicals damage and kill sperm, driving down its quality and its quantity.

The problem is so recognized that treatments are being explored. In one study out of Shanghai (*Chen, Hydrogen therapy may be a novel, safe and effective therapy for infertility patients with varicocele*), hydrogen gas and hydrogen-rich saline was used, to good effect. I don't know if I have varicocele or not, and that's not the point. The point is that a lot of men (?) all men (?) are under a burden of hydroxyl radicals, described by Dr. Morton Walker as "ubiquitous and highly injurious to health." I am supposing that these radicals were ubiquitous in my testicles, and highly injurious to my sperm health; and that DMSO cleared the place out like the new sheriff in town.

Are these hydroxyl free radicals "ubiquitous" in the female systems, too? Are they "highly injurious" to our ladies' health, also? It seems they are. Ruder's "Impact of oxidative stress on female fertility" tells us that, "oxidative stress is associated with decreased female fertility in animal and in-vitro models," although it remains unknown the extent of damage in women. But Agarwal's "Role of oxidative stress in female reproduction" assures us that oxidative stress "influences the entire reproductive lifespan of a woman," including, "a role in the pathophysiology of infertility."

Dr. Morton Walker links the use of DMSO's in the treatment of arthritis to its use in the treatment of cancer by way of free radicals. "Free radical pathology is an intricate part of virtually every metabolic dysfunction you can think of." Which would explain why DMSO seems to assist in every illness you can think of, as you see in the list above. Plus, at least in my own case, infertility.

Other actions of DMSO may have contributed to our success. Improved circulation, flushing of toxins from the insides of cells, and so on.

DMSO was never applied to my wife's reproductive parts. When you have a bicycle with two flat tires, it may be possible to get it moving if you can get only one tire inflated. But inflating both tires is surely better. In future, for other couples suffering infertility, it would be interesting to know the effects of DMSO treatment to both husband and wife, to both sets of gonads. I expect that the results could be even better.

If my theory about the mechanism of DMSO in curing infertility is correct, well and good. If incorrect, that's fine, too. I am not hard bound to any hypothesis of its modality. How it works is not nearly as important as the fact that it does work. That's how my family feels about it.

7
SAFETY STUFF

Is it safe? As we already know, it is safe enough to dump a million-dollar heart into a cooler full of the stuff. Safe enough to pop a couple of eyeballs into a thermos bottle of it. But let's reassure ourselves more.

The United States Food and Drug Administration (FDA) approves DMSO, right now, for medicinal use in the treatment of interstitial cystitis. This is a condition that causes scarring and shrinking of the bladder, and used to require major surgery, and sometimes the bladder's removal. In one study performed by Bruce Stewart, M.D., of the Cleveland Clinic Foundation, and Sheridan Shirley, M.D., of the University of Alabama, 213 patients were administered DMSO for interstitial cystitis. Of these patients, who had not responded well to traditional treatments, 75% achieved satisfactory relief, and 80% received "objective improvement in the endoscopic appearance of the disease, with improvement in bladder capacity."

Some state legislatures, frustrated that the FDA has not approved DMSO widely, have passed their own laws allowing it. Currently, I believe thirteen states have laws permitting doctors to prescribe DMSO for various conditions not allowed by the FDA.

The American College of Advancement in Medicine also seems to disagree with the FDA, as it has devised its own protocols for DMSO therapy.

Why does the FDA not approve DMSO for other conditions? I don't know. If you research this question, you will find that it seems to be more political than medical. I won't go into it. But there are a lot of good quotes by dissenting congressmen and senators who have looked into it. United States Senator Mark O. Hatfield (R-Ore.), for example, said of DMSO: "Since I have no scientific expertise, I cannot make an absolute statement that DMSO is indeed the wonder drug of our century, but every bit of evidence I encounter reinforces the premise that it is."

Dr. Morton Walker's last word on the subject is this. And I think these are good words by which to be guided: "As DMSO has been approved for use in interstitial cystitis by the FDA, DMSO is also legal in all fifty states for use in stroke, burns, arthritis, and for whatever other purpose the doctor deems appropriate." Himself a podiatrist, Dr. Walker uses DMSO in his practice for a great variety of foot conditions.

It is, in the United States, currently classified as an experimental drug for human use, and a prescription drug for veterinary use. By the way, we have mentioned million-dollar hearts. DMSO is also used on multi-million-dollar race horses! Experimentally in humans, DMSO has been administered topically, subcutaneously, intramuscularly, intraperitoneally, intravenously, orally, intrathecally, and by inhalation. It has been dropped into eyes and mucous membranes, and squirted into the urinary bladder. All with perfect safety.

In other parts of the world? A five-minute search finds that DMSO is used to treat urological disorders in Japan; gum disease in Poland and Bulgaria; scleroderma in Canada; shingles in Great Britain and Ireland; bursitis, tendinitis, arthritis, and "a whole host of disorders" in Germany and Austria; mental retardation, senility, rheumatic and cardiovascular disorders, chronic respiratory insufficiency, skin problems, and "other problems" in Chile; "a variety of disabilities" in Switzerland; and "the widest range of medical uses" in Russia. You can have fun finding more examples. In Europe and South America, doctors have been treating patients with DMSO for five decades. International symposia in Germany, the United States, and Austria have declared DMSO to be safe and effective.

The Physician's Desk Reference pronounces of DMSO, "There are no known contraindications."

Robert Herschler, chemist and discoverer of many pharmaceutical effects of DMSO, and Director of the DMSO Research Center, said the following, on the ABC-TV program, Good Morning America, in 1981: "...the toxicity of DMSO is very low. It's not true that it's dangerous. Compared to aspirin, DMSO is a much safer drug. People are killed taking aspirin; no one has ever been killed taking

DMSO." (Or to my knowledge harmed, I will add, beyond sometimes a little discomfort, of short duration.)

Another guest on the program was J. Richard Crout, M.D., Director of the FDA's Bureau of Drugs. Dr. Crout was defending the FDA's position on DMSO, but he had to admit: "It's really quite safe when put on the skin. I don't believe I would raise scare tactics about when people put it on and use it for a few days. Anybody who uses it for a month or more in doses of an ounce or more is getting into the unknown. There simply is not much experience with its toxicity there."

Much respect to Dr. Crout. I promise the Reader that I am not going to take you into that unknown territory, but let me remind you that it's not unknown to me. My friend's son drank 3 ounces of DMSO daily in orange juice, for about a year, and made a miraculous recovery from a crippling stroke!

Dr. Morton Walker reminds us that, "When fed to, injected into, or applied to the skin of animal laboratory subjects and human clinical subjects over periods of weeks, months, or years, there have been none or very few signs of any noxious response."

In toxicology there is something called the "median lethal dose" or LD_{50}. This is the number of milligrams (mg) of a substance per kilogram (kg) of body weight of the test subject, that it takes to kill half of the members of a tested population (the unlucky half). LD_{50} stands for Lethal Dose, 50 percent. Wikipedia has a good article on it.

You can't do this lethal testing on humans, so the information we have is for animals. Well now, The LD_{50} for aspirin swallowed, for monkeys, is 558 mg/kg. That's what it takes to kill half the monkeys that get into the aspirin bottle. The LD_{50} for DMSO swallowed, for monkeys, is 4,000 mg/kg. Therefore DMSO is 7 times safer than aspirin. That's when swallowed.

My friend's son weighed about 70 kg, and he took about 85,000 mg of DMSO daily in his orange juice. So he was swallowing about 1,214 mg/kg daily for months.

In the case of dunking laboratory mice into DMSO, the LD_{50} is 50,000 mg/kg. Mice survive complete immersion in up to 60% DMSO. Rats may be baptized in 80% DMSO, and they can enjoy repeated dippings in 60% solution three times a week for 26 weeks. So much for mice and rats. I am going to tell you, gentlemen, very frankly, that you may safely dunk your nuts into DMSO, as I have.

Humans experience, not always, but sometimes, a little reddening of the skin. About a third of persons feel a burning sensation. Smaller numbers of people report temporary skin roughness, itching, blistering, dermatitis, thickening, and scaling. According to Dr. Morton Walker, "None of these are toxic reactions but only side effects. Some of these effects are probably due to dehydration and removal of fats from the skin."

I have sometimes felt a mild itch, nothing more. My wife has used DMSO for non-reproductive purposes. Her skin is more sensitive than mine. She has experienced redness plus an "uncomfortable" itch, but her itch is relieved by sitting in front of an electric fan. We have found that using a lower concentration of DMSO, or a solution of DMSO and aloe vera, allows us to avoid the itch altogether.

Oh, and if you really slather it on, or drink a lot of it, some people get a bad body odor. But I have never experienced this, and I don't think anyone would, at the doses I used on myself.

Very important to note, "no cases of toxicity to the offspring of humans or animals from the skin applications of DMSO have been reported." Male and female rats, given DMSO orally at 50% strength, 5 grams per kilogram per day, for four days prior to mating, produced "no abnormality or infertility." I must wonder if they experienced better fertility, but that, it seems, was not looked for. The females were then fed DMSO throughout their gestation period. Their litters were born normal.

Entirely anecdotal, I know, but my own two DMSO babies were also born normal. Objectively, they are perfectly healthy girls, judged physically, mentally, and emotionally. Subjectively and truthfully, as a proud father, they are both happy, confident, sociable, comical, beautiful, and highly intelligent.

You can mainline DMSO. Real doctors do this. The LD_{50} for mice, when DMSO is shot into their veins, ranges from 3,800 to 8,900 mg/kg. The for LD_{50} monkeys is 4,000 mg/kg, the same as when they take the DMSO orally. Cats have the same intravenous LD_{50} as monkeys. Dogs are lower, at 2,500 mg/kg.

Ah, dogs. Dogs, rabbits, and pigs. These three animals, and only these three animals, seem to have a lower threshold for DMSO, and they can experience changes to their eyes: "refractive index changes in the lenses (not an opacity) of dogs, rabbits, and pigs." That is, DMSO, in large quantities, can make these three animals, and only these three animals, go a bit nearsighted. It changes But we are talking about large quantities and long durations: 5,000 mg/kg of DMSO for three months. To become "slightly nearsighted."

Let me tell you, I am a more than slightly nearsighted human. I am horrendously nearsighted, and have been since a child. I'm talking about your Coke-bottle glasses. That's me. Now even if this effect pertained to humans, I would gladly risk becoming a tiny bit more nearsighted than I am already, if it meant the difference between having and not having children. And now that my daughters are here, I would pluck my eyes out for them. I would grapefruit-spoon them out. But please be clear. This nearsightedness effect is observed only in dogs, rabbits, and pigs. The reader is, presumably, not a dog, or a rabbit, or a pig.

Has it been looked for specifically in humans? Yes. The University of Oregon Medical School subjected 32 human patients to an average dose of 30 grams of DMSO for from 3 to 20 months. That is a staggering amount. Thirty grams is 30,000 milligrams. One of the patients took 60 grams daily for 20 months: approximately 2 ounces. Examination by ophthalmologists discovered none of the lens-changing that would be seen in dogs, rabbits, or pigs. Zero. None.

The Cleveland Clinic, also, gave massive 30-gram doses to 44 patients, for as long as 23 months. None of these, either, experienced any lens changes.

Going back to my friend's son. He drank almost three times this amount, daily, for about a year. He did not experience any nearsightedness, either.

In Vacaville, California, 65 prison inmates volunteered to have DMSO in an 80% gel applied to their skin at 1,000 mg/kg for 14 days. There were no toxic effects.

A second group of 40 prisoners allowed themselves to be "coated with DMSO" for 3 months, also without toxic effect. As Dr. Morton Walker tells it: "Their eyes were examined with slit lamps, opthalmoscope, and tenometry; they were examined for lens refraction and visual fields, and underwent many blood, urine, liver, and other analyses. There were pulmonary function studies, neurological and other physical exams, and electrocardiogram studies. They were the most exhaustive series of toxicological studies that had been carried on for some time."

Here is the conclusion by the doctor in charge of the study, Richard D. Brobyn, M.D., of the Bainbridge Medical Center, Bainbridge Island, Washington: "A very extensive toxicology study of DMSO was conducted at three to thirty times the usual treatment dose in humans for three months. DMSO appears to be a very safe drug for human administration, and in particular the lens changes that occur in certain mammalian species do not occur in man under this very high prolonged treatment regimen. I am very glad to be able to present these data at this time so that we can permanently dispel the myth that DMSO is in any way a toxic or dangerous drug."

Also, I will remind you, human eyes are put into DMSO solutions for protection during storage and transport. A corneal transplant currently costs between $13,000 and $28,000, and the eyeballs are trusted to DMSO to keep them in the optimum condition.

About that last group of prisoners, Dr. Morton Walker estimates that they received at least 8.1 kg of DMSO over the 90 days (almost 18 lbs). That is 8,100 grams, or 8,100,000 milligrams. "Any other compound," says Dr. Walker, "such as sugar, salt, coffee, or tea taken in such huge quantities would kill the subject during this three-month period. Or, he would suffer from some severe metabolic problems. No so with the prisoners taking DMSO through the skin."

We could go on and on. It is hard to prove a negative, but I think this is one of those cases described by the logician Irving Copi: "In some circumstances it can be safely assumed that if a certain event had occurred, evidence of it could be discovered by qualified investigators. In such circumstances it is perfectly reasonable to take the absence of proof of its occurrence as positive proof of its non-occurrence."

As for me and my family, we have concluded that DMSO is safe. But please take, as your final anecdote, my wife. I finally did tell her about DMSO, of course. What I did, and so on. She was surprised but grateful. My wife, my biggest skeptic, looked into DMSO for herself. And she is no dummy. She graduated from an ivy league school. She's a good researcher. She worked in documents. Believe me, if my dear wife had found anything bad or worrisome about DMSO, I'd have heard about it. I'd *still* be hearing about it.

Little babies have viciously sharp little fingernails, and it often happens that they cut their precious faces. There are little protective baby mittens made especially to prevent this. Well, our baby girls, too, sometimes scratched or cut their faces. My wife's home remedy? Rub on a little DMSO. That's how convinced my wife is, after having examined the matter skeptically and thoroughly.

DMSO? Safe? Safe enough to rub on a baby's face. That's my wife's conclusion.

8
THE GREAT DAY

*T*he great day came. The day I would make family history. Also, I reckon, medical history. The calendar and the thermometer had determined it. It was D-Day.

Dunking Day.

"You went to school early." It was my wife on the phone.

"Yeah."

"You have work to do?"

"Yeah, yeah. A lot of work. And stuff. Yeah."

"Oh, okay."

"Yeah."

"Poor you."

"Yeah. No. I'm okay. I'm fine."

"Can I bring you some breakfast?"

"NO! No, thank you. I'm fine."

"You're sure?"

"Yes. Yes. Yes."

"Okay."

"Okay."

"So I'll come and pick you up later, then?"

"Yeah."

"Okay. I love you."

"I love you too."

"Bye."

"Bye."

We hung up, and I resumed dunking my balls in a cup of DMSO.

Isn't that a wonderful image? That's my first flight at Kitty Hawk. That's my Mr-Watson-Come-here-I-want-to-see-you. Me, naked from the waist down, straddling a stool, dunking my biscuits in a teacup. Perhaps one day, years from now, a group of grateful parents will erect a statue in my honour. I hope they will pose me just like that, dipping my cookies.

Unfortunately, the picture is not entirely historically accurate. I just imagined it that way because of the visual impact. In point of fact I was sitting on the very edge of a chair, and I was *daubing*, not dunking or dipping. D-Day properly stands for *Daubing Day*.

There is a 60 Minutes segment about DMSO. Mike Wallace did it, many years ago. I think it is still on YouTube. You can watch a doctor using a sort of cotton brush to apply DMSO to a patient. Dr. Morton Walker, in his book, explains how to apply DMSO carefully and correctly. Frankly, I didn't care about any of that. I just had my tub of DMSO gel open, and with one hand I was scooping it up and rubbing it onto my private parts. Rubbing it haphazardly and we may even say furiously. Now. There is the true historical, although less romantic, snapshot.

You will want to know how much DMSO did I use, and how many applications, and over what span of time, and so on. Unfortunately I did not weigh or measure out anything. Neither made nor kept records. Nothing like that. I wasn't doing science. I wasn't baking a cake. I was just desperately trying to make a baby.

Remembering back now though, I think I was at it for about a good 3 or 4 hours. I wanted to absorb as much DMSO as possible. I painted it on and rubbed it in until it was dry. Then I painted on the next coat, and the next, and so on, just like painting an old tool shed. Not exactly rocket science. Anyone could do it.

If I were a lady, I guess I would try to determine where my lady parts were, and paint directly over them. Ovaries, uterus. Oh, why not paint around the whole pelvis, too. It can't hurt. This is not advice. I'm saying that's what I would have done, if I were a lady.

If my recollection is correct, I was using a gel of DMSO + aloe vera. I won't tell you which brand in case they get mad. They might not want to be associated with me.

Now, dear Reader. You and I have always been very open with each other. Open and honest. I don't know if this next detail is important or not. It might be one ingredient in my success, so I will include it here. All of the time I was perched on the edge of my seat, applying more and more DMSO to myself, I was also fully aroused because I was studying pictures of attractive women. You see, I wanted my little Flying Zacchini Brothers to explode out of their cartoon circus cannon with as much force and excitement as possible. And I wanted as *many* Flying Zacchini Brothers as possible. Did studying pictures of attractive women help? I don't know. Perhaps. It is at least a factor to consider. Otherwise I wouldn't bring it up.

I was also watching the clock because I had to be dry and dressed when my wife came to get me. She did pick me up, and we drove to the fertility clinic.

"You were so busy this morning."

"Yeah. Yeah." I avoided her eyes.

Arrived at the clinic. Waited our turns. First I had to go into a room and make love to a petri dish, which I did. Then my wife had to go to her room. Then we were both finished. For my wife it was just another boring, expensive routine trip to the clinic. An appointment like any other. For me, it was a Great and Momentous Day.

Except it wasn't that because it turned out - my wife didn't get pregnant.

For my wife it was just another heart-wrenching, expensive disappointment. For me it was a Great and Momentous Disappointment. But not a deterrence. I still had full faith in my idea. So about one month later, or 28 days or whatever, it was D-Day, again. This time for real. The first one had been only a dress rehearsal.

I did the same thing. Got up early, snuck out of the house, studied pictures of attractive women, and saturated my apricots with DMSO. Got picked up. Drove to the fertility clinic. Made love to a another petri dish.

And that led to our daughter Matilda.

Now, I think I am a generous man, and a sharing man, but I give the fertility clinic not much credit, or none, for this breakthrough. Here is why.

The fertility clinic is a constant. Before DMSO came along, they had a perfect zero percent record, where we were concerned. Without DMSO, I have zero doubt that they would have come up zero again, like the zeroes they were, like the zeroes on all the money that I paid them. It doesn't mean that they were doing a bad job, necessarily. I don't mean to imply that. It's just that whatever they were doing wasn't working for us.

Enter DMSO. The first time, nothing. The second time, success. That's a fifty percent success record per trial, or a

100% success record for a two-month trial term. That's against the fertility record's zero.

Also. In the case of our second daughter, Florentina, we did not use the fertility clinic. We weren't even trying to have a baby. I wasn't even using DMSO.

Florentina, you see, confirms Matilda. Florentina confirms DMSO. Florentina confirms my original theory. Florentina, Florentina is the key. What was the only difference introduced between my epoch of sterility and my new epoch of dangerous fecundity? And what was the only constant between Matilda's conception and Florentina's? It was the DMSO. I recognize that this is not sufficient evidence for science, but I can hardly think of anything that would make me change my mind.

9
MATILDA IS BORN

Well, I wanted to tell my wife what I had done, but I couldn't do that. Not yet. She had to remain an unwitting participant for the time being. If anything went wrong with this pregnancy - if we lost the baby - or if the baby were born imperfect - who would be blamed? DMSO and me. Who might find themselves thrown out of the house and divorced? DMSO and me. So we still had to keep our secret for now, just DMSO and me.

Did I really tell no one? No one at all? No one at all. It was a long and tense time, and not only for me. Matilda wasn't bolted onto the uterine wall very strongly. There were fears that she might fall off. My wife was confined to bed for two months.

Toward the very end of the pregnancy, more trouble. Matilda didn't want to turn upside down. She liked sitting up. She was very stubborn. It looked like she was determined to be a breech birth. A lot more things can go wrong in a breech birth, and those things can be very bad. Our doctor decided that Matilda should be a caesarean baby, not a breech baby. Matilda was overruled.

The date and time were set. That's one advantage of a caesarean birth. You can schedule them. There is no water-breaking in movie theatres, and getting pulled over by police for speeding, and all of that bother. I was glad not to bother with that. I had bothers of my own, including of my own making.

I was confident that DMSO would not harm the baby. But you do have moments of doubt. Even if you have read and taken in all of the safety information, you do still have doubts. There was also our ages. We got married when I was 31. Add a 10 year delay from infertility... Well, we weren't young. There was higher risk of Down's syndrome, higher risk of heart defect, higher risk of everything, I suppose.

Matilda came out just perfect. She was the most beautiful little baby in the whole wide world forever, until her equally beautiful sister Florentina came and joined us four years later. My wife also did well. She made a quick and complete recovery. We were a family at last! And so we lived very happily and uneventfully ever after. Oh, I wish the story ended like this...

10
CALAMITY

After a woman gives birth, she is left with a big empty uterus. It can't just stay like that forever. It has to return to its normal size. So that's what it does. It shrinks back down to its regular size.

It turns out, though, a uterus doesn't want to do this. It acts like a crazed bobcat being stuffed into a burlap sack.

Imagine wrestling that bobcat, and one of its claws gets stuck in your lace curtain. If you thought that cat was freaking out before, now it is really going bananas. This, essentially, was the situation with my wife's uterus. It went bananas and tore the whole curtain rod down. In this analogy, the curtain rod represents one of the two main arteries that supplies blood to the uterus.

This happened about 10 days into our living happily ever after. My wife just started bleeding terribly. We took a fast taxi back to our little maternity hospital. I don't know why we called a taxi instead of an ambulance. Poor taxi man, we left him a bit of a mess.

They took my wife away. A nurse came and offered to put Matilda in the nursery. I didn't want to let her out of my arms, but the nurse said Matilda would be fine, and I would be able to help my wife more. I kissed Matilda goodbye, and sent her upstairs to be with the other babies. This was the correct decision because I was needed to help out. Boy, was I needed.

It was a Sunday or a national holiday or something. The hospital was running a skeleton crew. They were not prepared for us.

"Come here. Roll up your sleeves. Wash your hands and arms up to the elbow."

"What?"

"Your wife is in surgery."

"What?"

"We need your help."

"What?"

So I was press-ganged into assistant surgical nurse. They ushered me into a Hall of Horrors. There was my wife, lying lifeless-grey and naked on a stainless steel table. The table was running with blood. Our friendly obstetrician, lovely lady, was playing the part of an Aztec priestess who wanted to extract my wife's heart by way of the vagina.

"This is not good," our obstetrician said. "Your wife is bleeding very heavily."

"Yes," I said.

"I'm trying to find where all this blood is coming from."

"Yes, please."

"I can't stop the bleeding if I can't find where it's coming from."

"Right."

"I've ordered blood, but we're going to need a lot more blood."

"Oh?"

"It's coming out faster than I can get it in her."

"I see."

"And I have to make phone calls. As soon as we can get her stabilized for transport, she has to go to a major hospital."

"Right."

It seemed to me that our obstetrician looked more panicked that she should have been, and I was definitely calmer than I should have been, but she was understanding of the danger, and I was in shock.

I had several jobs all at once. I was to hold my wife's hand, and speak to her reassuringly. "It's okay, honey. You're looking great. Everything's going just fine," and other lies. With my other hand, I was to catch blood in a kidney pan. We had to catch all the blood to weigh it. With another hand I had to periodically hold up a blood transfusion bag. We had, in the end, three bags going in at one time.

Moments like these, when you're learning new skills, and telling lies to your dying wife, you lose track of time. I don't know how long we were at it. Maybe an hour. Often I was alone. The doctor kept going outside to make phone calls. To other hospitals. To the blood bank. To the ambulance.

My wife was sometimes barely conscious, mostly not. Twice I was sure she was dead. Hard to describe, but she deflated against the table. "There she goes," I thought. "She is really gone, and my last words to her were lies."

There was one other nurse besides me. She was in and out too. I remember she was being very meticulous about weighing the bottles of blood and keeping notes. Then she lined up the bottles of blood against the wall. By the end of it, those bottles contained slightly less than half my wife's blood.

"Good news," said the doctor coming back from one of her phone calls. "City Hospital can take her, and they have a new machine."

"Oh?"

"They got it last month. It's the only one in this region. And it's the only way to save your wife's life."

"I see."

"So let's get going."

"Okay." Again, shock is a wonderful thing. I sounded as if we'd just made plans to go for dinner and a movie.

So our obstetrician, my wife, and I piled into the ambulance and took off for City Hospital. My parents-in-law followed in their car, and beat us. Along the way my wife deflated once or twice more. Just deflated into her stretcher.

New hospital, new doctor, new machine. I sat on a stool opposite the doctor. My wife's parents stood behind me.

"So we have two options," the new doctor said to my wife's mom and dad and me. "Number One, the safest thing, and the easiest thing, is to perform a hysterectomy. We remove the whole uterus. That way we can stop the bleeding for sure.

"The other option, Number Two, we can try out our new nuclear imaging machine, and try to find the hemorrhage and repair it. But it is risky as she is still bleeding."

"Do Number One," my wife's parents told him. "Do Number One."

"I'm sorry," said the doctor. "This is the husband's decision, not yours."

My wife's parents' eyes burned like lasers into the back of my head.

"Couldn't you remove the uterus, and fix it, and put it back in?" I asked.

"No. A hysterectomy is irreversible."

"I see." Oh, the heat of those laser eyes! "Well, with Number Two, what are the chances it goes well? What are the risks?"

"I can't say."

"Oh." The back of my head was feeling very hot indeed. I think it was smoking.

"Mr. Mountebank, whichever you decide, you have to decide quickly."

"Yes. Well, my wife and I, we want to to have another baby, if we can."

"One is enough!" my parents-in-law said. "You're lucky enough to have one. One is enough!"

The doctor shushed them, and reminded me that my wife was still bleeding to death.

"Do Number Two," I told him.

My parents-in-law deflated. Their lasers went out.

The nuclear imaging team assembled. They looked like college kids. Their chief was a cute young girl. They started pumping radioactive fluid into my wife as I supervised and made sure they knew what they were doing.

"We're going to start. You have to leave now, sir."

"Yes."

"Come on," my in-laws said.

"Yep, I'll be right there."

"Sir," said the cute girl chief. "We'll handle it from here. But you have to wait outside."

I took my wife's hand one last time. She was conscious. I lied to her once more, that she was perfectly safe, and so on. Then I left with my parents-in-law.

We started down the corridor. Damn it, I forgot to tell her I loved her.

"Hengist, come back!"

Too late. I smashed through the doors into the nuclear room again. The cute chief looked surprised to see me back so soon.

I grabbed my wife's hand and told her I loved her.

"I love you too."

"Thank you for our baby. Thank you for everything."

"Thank you, too."

"Bye."

"Bye."

11
FLORENTINA IS BORN

That was an awkward time, waiting in the waiting room with my parents-in-law. They thought I was stupid and wrong for choosing Option Two. And maybe I was, maybe I was. We would have to wait and see.

The college kids found the rupture. They patched it up. They saved the day. They saved my wife. They saved her criminally-insane bobcat uterus. I had made the correct decision after all. Maybe not the smart decision, but anyway the lucky decision.

We saw my wife in the I.C.U. and lied to her some more, and then went back to the little maternity hospital to pick up Matilda. Poor thing, she'd been in the nursery all day, separated from her mother. From me, too.

"You're free to take her home," the obstetrician told me. "But it will be hard for you, taking care of her all by yourself. If you like, you can leave her here while your wife recovers."

My parents-in-law thanked the doctor, and accepted her kind offer.

"Do you think it's dangerous if I take her home?" I asked.

"No, not dangerous. You can do it. But it will be hard for you, alone."

"Then I'm taking her home."

"Very good. Then I'll get her ready to go."

My parents-in-law complained. I couldn't do it, they said.

I said my daughter was not a piece of baggage to be stowed. She was my baby daughter, and I was taking her home.

"But the hospital can care for her better than you."

"I can care for her. I am her father. Hospitals are for sick people. This baby isn't sick. I'm taking her home."

"Oh, please, Hengist Mountebank! Please reconsider!" they said.

"I'll make you a deal," I said. "I'll take her home to my house and take care of her all by myself. Or I'll take her home to your house, and you can help me take care of her. But I am not leaving her here. I am taking her home, one way or another."

"Ah. Well. Then let's all go home to our house."

"Super. Thank you."

Emotions were frazzled all around, but we were okay. I loved my in-laws, and they loved me. And we all loved my wife, and we all loved baby Matilda, so we all pulled together. Taking care of a newborn baby *is* hard, but we did just fine. And then, at last, my wife came home and took over. We all stayed with my in-laws a little longer, and then my family went back to our own house.

Family. We were a family at last.

I went with my wife for a follow-up visit.

"You must never get pregnant again," said our obstetrician.

"Yes, Ma'am."

"You." She wagged her finger in my face like she was Sister Mary-Apocalypse. "You must never, ever make her pregnant, ever again. Ever."

"Yes, Ma'am."

"She cannot have this again. She cannot take it. She cannot do it."

"Yes, Ma'am."

"She will not endure it. She will not survive next time."

"Yes, Ma'am."

"You will kill her."

"Yes, Ma'am."

"Your penis will kill her."

"Yes, Ma'am."

"You will murder her with your penis if you make her pregnant again."

"Yes, Ma'am."

"Do you understand me?"

"Yes, Ma'am."

She lowered her finger but not her eyes. She glared and glared.

"You were very, very lucky this time."

"Yes, Ma'am."

"You will not be that lucky next time. Okay?"

"Okay."

Several more times the obstetrician impressed upon me the supreme importance of never making my wife pregnant again. But I thought she pressed too much. I already knew we would never be back here again. For several reasons.

We were hopelessly infertile.

I was putting away my DMSO forever.

My nursing wife didn't feel very sexy.

My wife's naked body didn't feel very sexy to me; it felt more scary.

I think I had PTSD. I had dreams and hallucinations of gushing blood.

After years of sex on command, we both felt kind of sexed-out.

Sex without any reproductive purpose felt depressing.

Matilda completed us.

Our sleeping arrangements were prohibitive.

And so on. It seemed that my wife and I would live, from now on, like celibates.

Then, when Matilda turned two years old, my wife stopped nursing. She got feeling like her old self again. To me she started looking like her old self again. I stopped thinking of gushing blood and death. We got together intimately again, but still very infrequently and with precautions.

Very infrequently. As elsewhere in this story, I was not taking records. There are no diaries to consult. But again, for the sake of total honesty, I will hazard that we were intimate, over the next two years, fewer than ten times. And always taking precautions. Except once.

"I'm pregnant," she said, looking dazed.

"Wow."

"Yeah."

"What do you want to do?"

"What do *you* want to do?"

"I want to have it if you do."

"I want to have it if I can."

"Yeah."

"Yeah."

So we found ourselves back facing Sister Mary-Apocalypse.

"Congratulations," she sighed. "But you cannot have your pregnancy here. You are too high risk. You must do it all at City Hospital, beginning to end."

That was a scary nine months. I feared for my wife, and we both feared for the baby. Her cantankerous old uterus now had only half its original blood supply. Would half be enough to support a baby? No one promised it would be. No one was sure. We talked it over and agreed that we would love it and care for it no matter how it came out.

My fears were mostly relieved around month six or seven. We were being very closely monitored all the way. We had a lot of doctor visits and ultrasounds. On this particular day I was sharing a lot of worries. I'd been doing too much reading on high-risk pregnancies. I had too many monsters in my head. We were all looking up at the ultrasound screen. Little Florentina was there, sitting in profile, paying us no mind. Then the most amazing thing.

Florentina slowly turned to face the camera, looked right into it, and gave us a thumbs-up.

"You see, Papa?" said the doctor. "She's telling you, Don't worry. Everything is fine in here. Everything is going to be just fine."

Doctor, wife, Matilda - everyone was laughing at me. So I had to laugh too, and stop worrying.

Baby Florentina was right. She *was* fine. She came out with the most perfectly symmetrical and extremely pronounced mohican hairstyle, which she rocked for all her first year.

But after the delivery, on a follow-up visit, the doctor was very firm with us.

"You must never, ever be pregnant again."

"We know."

"No. You don't understand. You don't know how close you came."

"What, last time? This time?"

"This time."

The doctor explained. When he sliced open my wife to extract her precious cargo, he saw something that he had never seen before.

As he peeked inside the abdomen, he did not see the uterus. He saw only flat-nosed Florentina staring back at him. The uterus had stretched as thin and transparent as Saran wrap. It was barely holding together. And Florentina was pressing with her hands, and pushing with her legs, and doing acrobatics on that weak and sorry Saran wrap.

"It was stretched way beyond its limit. There's no telling how much longer until it burst. Maybe minutes."

"If it burst, that wouldn't be good," I guessed.

"It would not have been good," the doctor agreed. "We could have lost them both. It's damned lucky that we got in there when we did. You are very lucky."

"Yes," I said, hugging Matilda on my lap, and looking at Florentina and my wife. "Yes, we sure are."

My wife and I had gone again to the very limit of life and pushed and kicked on it, like Florentina. We almost met our LD_{50} of making babies - twice. My wife, she didn't just come to Death's door. She knocked on it, opened it, and stepped inside Death's foyer. That damned door almost shut on her, leaving me outside and alone.

This is another reason why I won't give you advice, and I will not urge you to do what I did. You might end up severely injured, or dead, or widowed. You might end up with a severely handicapped child. Or you might come out with a happy, healthy family. I don't know. It's a gamble. In my own family's case, we were lucky. We dodged the disasters. It was worth it, every bit.

12
CONCLUSION

Life is a frail thing. Frail and desperately precious. How have I come close to losing mine? In a blizzard, my father losing control of the car in a rock cut, and sliding into the way of an oncoming semi. Playing hockey, and falling through the ice. Twice. Being hit by a car, and sailing over two lanes of traffic, into a concrete divider. (My laced-up shoes continued for two more lanes.) A mad dog, an inch away from my femoral artery. A wall falling on my head, almost crushing my temple. Those are a few.

And then a near-infinity of events that could have, or should have, prevented me. On my matrilinear line, without even going far back, my great-grandmother, as a young girl, half-drowned in a lake. She had an out-of-body experience. Her husband, my great-grandfather, died from "valvular heart disease, mitral stenosis and regurgitation, with nephritis as contributing condition" when my grandmother was three. The day of the funeral, my grandmother, thinking to be helpful, went out to milk the cow. Approached it from the wrong side, and BANG got kicked in the head, cracking it.

My dad, when he was seven. His parents, and all 10 children, were immigrating to Canada from Holland. Everyone needed shots. My dad drew some kind of short straw. One of his shots gave him meningitis. He was comatose, and the condition was 100% fatal. The family, having sold off all, was possessionless and homeless; now they were going to miss their ship, and my dad was going to die. The Dutch doctors had an experimental drug. Shall we try it? They tried it. My dad recovered. He was the first-ever patient to live. You can read about the case in old medical journals.

Matilda and Florentina. They would not be here if I hadn't been reading about the use of DMSO in organ transplantation. And if God himself hadn't moved me to make the connection. Now that we have them, I am a bit obsessive about keeping them safe and alive. We do our best, but illnesses and accidents do happen. It was only a few months ago that I was living in the hospital with Matilda. She had pneumonia and was drowning in her fluids. Attached to an oxygen mask for a week. That was hard. Florentina fell on a windowsill - on her teeth - detaching her top right incisor. The dentist was able to push it back into position, and it took root again. Thank God, we get out of most of these jams. Most of us do. Some of us don't. Here are some real headlines from recent weeks.

Girl, 4, falls off swing, breaks neck.

Two-year-old has arms, legs amputated because of mystery illness.

Rape of girl, 7, in a restaurant toilet.

"Happy, bubbly" 2-year-old boy killed in hit-run smash.

Landslide kills 8, victims mostly children.

Police find body of missing 3-year-old. Tortured, raped.

Six-month-old boy kidnapped, burned to death, found near railway tracks.

Of course I always knew that such things happened. I knew. But now I *know*.

I am, compared to most other dads, overprotective. Sorry, but that's how I am. I don't even think it is overprotective. I think most other dads are *under*protective. I feel about my daughters as Major General William H. Rupertus felt about his rifle, and no one says he was overprotective about his rifle! If I may borrow from his Rifleman's Creed: *These are my daughters; there are many like them, but these ones are mine. My daughters are my best friends. They are my life. I must master them as I must master my life. Without me, my daughters are useless. Without my daughters, I am useless.* And so on.

Delayed parenthood has made me, in almost every way, a better father. I treasure my daughters more. I thank God for them more. I know how unique and irreplaceable they are. I am more patient with them. I am non-violent. I spend more time with them, and enjoy their companionship more. Diapers, vomit, midnight vigils, spills, breakage, crayon on the wall? Buddy, I've bottled up half of my wife's blood to be here, to enjoy this. Parents who complain about parenting on Facebook - I hate them, and I pity them.

Delayed parenthood has also, I believe, made my wife and me better partners. We know better how much we need each other. We respect each other better. We love each other more. We're battle-hardened. Again, I have never held my buddy's guts at Passchendaele. Never carried my buddy across a Normandy Beach. No. Not my buddy. My *wife*.

I titled this book, I told you, after a line from the song, *This Woman's Work*. If you would do me a favour, please watch that music video. The montage sequence that begins around 2:40.

That is my wife, and my wife is my hero. She put her life on the line for our daughters and me, out of love.

I ended the last chapter saying that everything we went through was worth it. Let me be more frank. As far as my wife and I are concerned, if only Matilda and Florentina were here with me in the house, asleep in their beds upstairs, it would have been worth it. If only Matilda, still worth it. That's how much we wanted these babies. We felt that they deserved their turn at life, and we both (theoretically) but mostly my wife (in practice) were comparatively expendable. Yeah, easy for me to say. But let me tell you, it wasn't so easy for my wife to do.

Thank you, Wife, for laying down your life.

Thank you, God, for giving it back, multiplied.

13
YOUR BAKER'S DOZEN

*B*onus story. In this story I almost died. But first I have to go back about a year before that. I was all alone, washing dishes. Plates, cups, cutlery, and finally the nice big wine glasses. Nice big Burgundy globes. Like an idiot I had my hand inside one.

I have tried, until now, not to give advice. But please take my advice this time and never do that because...

[*Crack*]

The glass cracked and sliced my hand.

I held up my hand to assess the damage. It looked fine. A nice clean cut and no blood. No blood for about 1 second. Then there was a Burgundy velvet curtain.

This was not a typical cut. A little Band-Aid would not work. The sheer volume of blood would wash it away. I needed stitches. Or staples. Or something.

I had read or heard somewhere that Cayenne pepper is good for bleeding. Actually, I had heard it was good for heart attacks. I heard that old-time country doctors sometimes carried Cayenne pepper in their medical bags. Because sometimes, when someone is having a heart attack out in the countryside, you don't have time to wait for the ambulance. So these old guys would order the farmwife to make a cup of hot water, then they'd dump a good spoonful of Cayenne pepper in it, and force the farmer with the heart attack to drink it. And apparently this can stop a heart attack in its tracks. Also it's good for high blood pressure, which I have. So I was in the habit of drinking Cayenne pepper tea once or twice a week. With a bit of honey it isn't so bad.

Well, that's why I had a little spice jar of Cayenne pepper in my cabinet, for high blood pressure and heart attacks. But I'd also heard that Cayenne pepper is good for unstoppable bleeding. I got the little spice jar, opened it, and sprinkled the red powder on my hand. The blood stopped.

All right, fast-forward about a year. It was a fine autumn day. I was all by myself again, ransacking an abandoned hospital - with the owner's permission of course, when suddenly...

I didn't know what hit me. I came to on the floor. My head rang like a bell. My glasses were gone. I pushed myself up. I was bleeding. How much? A lot. From where? From my face. From my nose. I stumbled over to a mirror. Leaned in for a good, hard, squinty look. A chunk of my nose bridge was missing. I was looking at a gap of raw flesh and cartilage.

Back to the scene. I saw what had happened. An unfastened backboard, basically a wall, fell on me. I knew that this fallen wall was the culprit because there, stuck to the edge of it, was my nose meat and nose gristle. I found my glasses, pocketed them, and exited the premises, taking care to lock up behind me.

This was only a block from my office, so I headed back there. The front of my shirt was all blood-soaked. I looked like a one-man zombie apocalypse.

Long wait for the elevator up to my third-floor suite. In my sunny front room would be my good buddy Bob McCloset, working on his computer. (Bob was still my buddy in those halcyon days. I still had my life savings. My house was not in jeopardy of seizure. I had no debts. No one had ever sexually assaulted me... Those were good times.)

Well, there was Bob McCloset, all right, in my best room, existing on my charity. He had his back to me and his headphones on. I tapped him on the shoulder. He turned around and jumped almost out of his skin.

"Dude, what happened to you!?"

"I got hit by a wall."

"Hit by a car?"

"Hit by a *wall*."

"Oh, man, I think your nose is broken, dude."

"I know."

"You're bleeding a lot."

"I know."

"I'll drive you to the hospital."

"I don't have time for that."

"Dude, you need stitches."

"There's nothing to stitch back together. The nose meat is gone."

"Dude!" Bob McCloset wretched.

"Come here, I need your help." I took him to the kitchen. Prepared a chair for myself, and put the jar of Cayenne pepper in his hands. "I'm going to cover my eyes with my hands. You dump this on my nose."

"Dude, are crazy? What? Why?"

"Do it."

"Dude, it'll hurt like crazy."

"Do it."

Actually, Cayenne pepper on a wound does not burn. It gives a warm sensation, but I wouldn't call it painful. If anything, it seems to have an anaesthetizing effect. The bleeding stopped, as I knew it would.

"That's amazing," said my trusted buddy Bob.

"Yes. Cayenne pepper is amazing."

"Now I'll take you to the hospital."

"No. I don't have time. I have a full afternoon."

"But dude, you need a doctor."

"For what?" I was looking in a mirror, scraping away blood and excess Cayenne pepper from the sides of my nose and face, and wiping clean an area so a Band-Aid could stick. "What's a doctor going to do? There's nothing to stitch back together. That section of nose is gone. I'd just be wasting the doctor's time and mine. There." I had got the Band-Aid on my nose, and my glasses on top of the Band-Aid. "That's pretty good, I think."

"Dude, you're crazy."

"This will be fine," I reassured him as I sponged more blood and pepper off my face. For I was preparing to put on some DMSO.

When I got home that evening I took off the regular old Band-Aid, and put on one of those fancy gel-type Band-Aids that you stick on and leave on forever. The Cayenne pepper I left in the wound. I did not wash out the wound.

Daily, or as often as I remembered to do it, I rubbed DMSO around the Band-Aid perimeter. I couldn't get it on the wound directly. That was fine. As we know, DMSO gets into the bloodstream and goes where it needs to go.

My nose made a complete recovery. I tell people this story now, and take off my glasses, and show them my nose.

"Where?" they say. "*There?*"

The bridge of my nose is grown back. First it covered with a scab, and then skinned over, but there was still a section of missing material. That gap lifted up and filled in. The bridge of my nose is complete and smooth. There is only a 1-centimeter patch where the skin is a little lighter, and a little more wrinkly when I wrinkle my nose at certain persons. If you push down lightly there, it's puffy and soft. It doesn't feel like the bridge of a nose because the cartilage is missing. But just looking from the outside, you'd never know that. And with my glasses on, it's totally invisible.

If my head had been turned a few degrees to the right when the wall hit, it would have hit me in the left temple. As it had enough weight and force to take out a section of nose and knock me down and out, it surely would have shattered my temple like an eggshell. It would have killed me. That would have been a terrible day for me, and also for my friend Bob Conman, for a parasite cannot live without its host. I only lost a piece of nose, but that gave me another opportunity to test the wondrous healing powers of DMSO. So there is one more story about this amazing substance to which I owe my daughters and - my nose.

14
VOLUNTEER STUDY

I wish I had a stronger pitch than, "Hey, man. I rubbed this stuff on my balls, and it worked for me." I wish I were able to say, "Hey, man. I and 370 other people rubbed this stuff on our balls, and it worked for 80 percent of us."

In a future edition of this book, I would like to have more data than just mine. As much data as possible. Here's where you come in.

If you independently happen to get the same idea as me, to rub DMSO on your balls and/or ovaries to assist with conceiving a baby, please let me know how it goes. I will keep records, and incorporate the information in this book's second edition. Then again, if you give me enough information, it might deserve a whole new book. Let's see.

I don't want to hear from quitters. If you try DMSO one time and then give up on it, I won't include you in this informal study. You would be skewing the results. Remember my parents-in-law, who sprayed colloidal silver on Blackie's ear one time, and quit. Stopping there, it might be recorded that the colloidal silver failed. Whereas it only required one more application, and the skin cancer got better.

Again, please remember. I did not beget Matilda on my first try. I begat her on my second try. So I think we have to be fair to DMSO, and fair to the hypothesis (in my own mind tested and proven) that it can resolve at least some cases of infertility.

What is fair? I don't know. I'll suggest that you keep up with it for at least 6 months before you report that it didn't work. I think that is a fair enough trial. Twelve months would probably be fairer because infertility is usually only diagnosed when a couple hasn't managed to conceive after a year of trying.

Whether you are successful after any time, or unsuccessful after at least 6 months, I wish that you would write to me in as much detail as possible. If you spin a really good yarn, perhaps I will reproduce your letter in its entirety. Without your name or identifying details, of course.

I would especially like to know the following.

How many applications did it take before a successful conception?

How long did you try to conceive before using DMSO?

Was the cause of your infertility ever explained to you?

What are your ages?

Who used the DMSO? The man? The woman? Both?

What brand of DMSO did you use?

What form of DMSO? Liquid? Gel?

How exactly did you apply it?

How often?

How long before coitus (or clinical procedure) did you apply it?

Did you apply it only topically?

What side-effects, if any, did you experience?

What side-benefits, if any, did you experience?

What other treatments, if any, were you using?

And anything else that you feel is important or interesting.

Please send letters to me at hengistmountebank@gmail.com.

And again, if this book has helped you, and you would like to support my work and message, you may like to become a regular patron of mine, on Patreon: patreon.com/HengistMountebank

Or you might like to make a one-time donation at Paypal: Paypal.me/HengistMountebank

One or more of these links may advise you that your payment is going to a certain person whose name rhymes with "Vile Drink." Don't be afraid. Everything is correct. This person is my trusted lifelong, er, private secretary.

Thank you.

AFTERWORD

And once more, thank you for reading this book. Whatever interest you have in infertility, and wherever you go from here, please go with my blessing.

My deepest gratitude to Dr. Morton Walker, on whom I have leaned heavily for chapters six and seven. Everyone should buy his book, DMSO Nature's Healer. It is much better than this book, and belongs on every bookshelf. Along with a jar of DMSO.

I myself keep six large bottles of the stuff on the top shelf of the closet in my study. With instructions for my wife on its use. It is not to be opened except in dire emergency, and I mean life-threatening emergency. We didn't even open it last summer when I was barbecuing barefoot, like a fool, and stepped on a burning piece of charcoal. The charcoal stuck to my foot and wouldn't shake loose, and it burned into my flesh as I dance-hopped over to the garden hose. No, not even that second-degree barbecuing of my foot was enough to make me open my emergency cache. I used comfrey oil instead, and my foot healed up just fine. "Amazing," is the word Dr. T. used.

Very well. Enough of Uncle Hengist's old man's ramblings. I have brought you my information. I have tried to make it as clear as I can. And although it's a gloomy and difficult topic, I have tried to be as human and hopeful and encouraging and positive as I can, without being flippant.

Our theme is time-sensitive. I have hurried to write it, and now I am hurrying to bring it to market. Mistakes, surely, have been made and not caught. I will try to catch them in a second edition.

This book was longer by almost a third, but I cut out a lot. Some might wish I had cut even more. I suppose it could be shorter, but then it would be a pamphlet or a booklet, not a book. The USPS defines a book as "a bound publication having 24 or more pages." So if I wanted to be saucy, I could say this book is almost double length! No. It's a slim little book, but it's a book. I hope you get your money's worth and more. I hope you get about a million billion trillion times your money's worth!

This Woman's Work contains this plea:
Give me these moments back
Give them back to me
Give me that little kiss
Give me your hand

The singer is looking backwards at the past. I want to take these words and turn them around, and point them into the future. *Your* future. Now they are your words, aren't they? You want these moments with your child. You want to have that little kiss. You want to take that tiny hand. This is your prayer, and mine also, for your sake. Therefore I end by asking the Lord God to use this poor book and make it a blessing to you.

Hengist Mountebank
January, 2019

Made in the USA
Columbia, SC
24 July 2023